Nutrition Management for Children with Attention Deficit Hyperactivity Disorder

Wendy Phillips, MS, RD, CNSC, CLE, FAND

DEDICATION

This book is dedicated to my son, Austin Phillips, who inspired me to write this book as we have learned about ADHD together as a family. It is also dedicated to my husband Marcus and son Tyler, who have supported me over countless hours of reading research and talking with children and adults with ADHD, and have allowed our couch to be literally covered with research articles for more nights than I can count!

I also acknowledge and appreciate the excellent work referenced in this book that has been done, and continues to be done, by scientists and researchers in many areas related to nutrition and ADHD. Children's lives are made better by the work that you are doing.

I also would like to express love and appreciation for the many wonderful teachers my sons have had over the years, with a special dedication to Mrs. Julie Galland for her support and guidance for this book.

CONTENTS

FOREWORD

Thank you for choosing to read this book! As a mother, my hope is that you will read the stories about our family's adventure of living and coping with ADHD to learn strategies that will help as you live with the disease yourself or someone close to you who has this disease. I hope you laugh, but mostly you'll probably think to yourself "I'm so glad it isn't just me!"

As a registered dietitian nutritionist (RDN), I hope that you'll learn nutrition strategies to maximize management of ADHD, whether or not you choose to complement that with medication and/or behavioral therapy.

I start out the book with a brief overview of ADHD: how it is diagnosed, the underlying etiology of the disease, and the common treatments. Then, I share nutrition research and management strategies. I'll share stories about my son throughout the book, because it helps to translate the research into real life, every day practical terms that actually work with kids! Sometimes I will use big words and medical terms, but I will always try to translate that into plain English for those non-healthcare professionals who may be reading this book.

So let's get started with the Introduction…which of course is an introduction to my son!

1 INTRODUCTION

Austin is the second of two boys God blessed us with and is now 13 years old. He has always been amazing at any sport he tried – football, soccer, basketball, baseball, hockey, ice skating, anything! He climbed on everything he could anywhere we went. And we knew from a very young age that he had a brilliant mind that could figure out science, building, engineering, math, and similar subjects almost effortlessly. He has always been the child who questioned the why and what and how of everything -- wanting to know everything from why clouds look different from one day to the next to the function of every piece in an electronic gadget to the physics behind making a hanging bridge...and the list could go on and on! We relied heavily on science books for kids to help answer his questions.

His third grade teacher encouraged us to get him tested for what she thought at the time was anxiety disorder, but the school district wouldn't test him because it wasn't affecting his grades or other children around him. We sought independent testing at a children's psychology center, and were blessed to get him entered in a research study that included 8 intensive sessions of testing for any disorder related to attention or anxiety. Through this testing, they measured his gross and fine motor movements with actigraphs (activity monitors) on his ankles and wrists, and tested him using many different techniques such as interactive computer games, attention tests, and other scientifically validated methods. They tested him for intellectual ability as well as for any disorders related to attention deficit behaviors. We completed many questionnaires based on his actions at home, and his teachers completed the same questionnaires for his behavior at school. Ultimately, he was diagnosed as a genius with Attention Deficit Hyperactivity Disorder (ADHD) at the age of 10. I can't even put into words the relief that my husband and I had when we got the final report from the psychologist: 1. Our son was not suffering from anxiety or depression, as we had feared, and 2. He had a real disease that we could address.

It didn't hurt at all of course to confirm our suspicions – that he is a genius! We debated on whether we should even tell him that – because children sometimes can either brag about their abilities or use that kind of knowledge to think they can do the bare minimum and still get by. We did end up telling him, but told him not to share this information with his friends. Rather, he needs to appreciate and utilize his God-given talents to help others and utilize his intelligence to make a difference in the world.

Throughout this book I will share stories and information about how we and the teacher knew to get him tested, with the hopes that you'll know if you should also get your child tested. Of course, not everyone will have access to the extensive testing that we had through the University center, but your family physician or psychologist can recommend the appropriate method for testing.

2 DIAGNOSING ADHD

This chapter is very important to understanding a lot of the information that I will share in this book. You will need to have a basic understanding of the etiology (causes) of ADHD to understand the nutrition research for specific nutrients. You need to know the symptoms associated with ADHD to understand the nutrition-related behavior management techniques we will discuss. You may want to refer back to this chapter periodically as you read the other chapters!

Diagnosis

The Diagnostic and Statistical Manual of Mental Disorders – 5th edition (DSM-5)[1] is used throughout the world for the formal diagnosis of mental and behavioral disorders, including ADHD. Table 1 includes an overview of much of the diagnostic classification for ADHD; healthcare professionals should read the entire section of the DSM-5 manual for more detailed information. There are three presentations (types) of ADHD:

1) combined,

2) inattentive, and

3) hyperactive/impulsive.

Children have different degrees of severity, ranging from mild to severe symptoms. A commonly asked question is "what is the difference between ADHD and ADD

(Attention Deficit Disorder)?" The answer is as simple as the names imply: People with ADD are not hyperactive like people with ADHD and are considered in 2nd category of "inattentive".

Table 1. Diagnostic classification for ADHD from the Diagnostic and Statistical Manual of Mental Disorders – 5th edition[1] (not a complete list).

✓ Inattention and/or hyperactivity-impulsivity interferes with development or day-to-day life
✓ Several symptoms present prior to age 12 years
✓ Several symptoms present in two or more settings (e.g. at home, school, or work; with friends or relatives; in other activities)
✓ Clear evidence that the symptoms interfere with social, academic or occupational functioning

While it is true that people with ADHD are considered hyperactive, it does not necessarily mean gross motor movements such as running around the classroom or getting up and down and out of their seats frequently. The hyperactivity may be more of a fine motor movement such as slight but nearly continuous hand or feet movements, fidgeting, or tics such as rapid eye movement or grunting. While completing routine actions like tying shoes or writing, these children may include extra movements that distract from completion of the task. Different people manifest ADHD in different ways and different degrees; stigmatizing or stereotyping children and adults with ADHD is counterproductive and can be hurtful.

For children and adolescents younger than 17, six or more of the symptoms listed in Table 2 must have been present for at least six months in at least two different settings (such as at home or at school) and must occur by the age of 12[1]. Five or more of these symptoms are required for diagnosing older adolescents and adults. Symptoms commonly thought to be associated with ADHD in children, such as gross (visible) movement and hyperactivity, are less common with adults. However, problems usually persist with poor planning, impulse control, inattentiveness, and restlessness that can lead to a lower quality of life for an adult with ADHD if not managed correctly[2].

Table 2. Behaviors associated with ADHD

Some examples of inattentive types of behaviors that parents or teachers may notice:
✓ Failing to give close attention to details or making careless mistakes in schoolwork, at work, or with other activities. *Many children will occasionally forget to put their name on their paper; kids with ADHD will often forget details like that or will not fully read a question or a book in order to truly understand the assignment.*
✓ Often has trouble holding attention on tasks or play activities. *These children may often bounce from one activity to another, even if it is something active like playing a sport. Teachers and parents often give multiple-part instructions for assignments; it may be difficult for a child with ADHD to pay attention to all of the details of the instructions.*
✓ Often does not seem to listen when spoken to directly. *May also have difficulty maintaining eye contact.*
✓ Often does not follow through on instructions and fails to finish schoolwork, chores, or duties in the workplace (e.g., loses focus, side-tracked). *I noticed that we could only give my son one instruction at a time, and once he completed that task, we would give him the next instruction. For example, we couldn't tell him to*

put the laundry away, clean the bathroom sink, and clean his bedroom, because he would only do one of the chores and then lose track and forget about the other items.

✓ Often has trouble organizing tasks and activities. *We learned to give him specific instructions – instead of saying "clean your room" we would say "clean your desk so that nothing is left on the top surface". Then, when that was completed, we would give him the next specific instruction like "hang up your clothes in the closet".*

✓ Often avoids, dislikes, or is reluctant to do tasks that require mental effort over a long period of time (*such as schoolwork or homework*).

✓ Often loses things necessary for tasks and activities (*e.g. school materials, pencils, books, tools, wallets, keys, paperwork, eyeglasses, cell phones*).

✓ Is often easily distracted and forgetful in daily activities. *Often, by the time Austin had climbed the stairs to his bedroom he had forgotten the task we gave him.*

Examples of hyperactivity and impulsivity behaviors may include:

✓ Often fidgeting with or tapping hands or feet, squirming in seat. *Several parents have told me their child adds extra movements to almost everything they do, like setting the table or cleaning their room or getting dressed.*

✓ Leaving seat in situations when remaining seated is expected, *such as leaving the dinner table at home or at a restaurant.*

✓ Children will often run about or climb in situations where it is not appropriate whereas adolescents or adults may feel restless. *I have had many children with ADHD climb on window sills or chairs while in my office; other children sit in the chair but constantly move their fingers or legs.*

✓ Often unable to play or take part in leisure activities quietly. *Children may play a board game but talk*

> *continuously throughout it.*
> ✓ Is often "on the go" acting as if "driven by a motor". *Many kids will act like this during exciting situations, such as at a birthday party or amusement park; children with ADHD may act like this in more settings and at more times, even if in a routine place or event.*
> ✓ Is known to talk excessively and blurt out an answer before a question has been completed. *Such as my son spelling the words out loud for the classroom spelling test.*
> ✓ Often has trouble waiting his/her turn. *This is a reason that many kids with ADHD have trouble making or keeping friends. Standing in line is especially difficult!*
> ✓ Often interrupts or intrudes on others (e.g., butts into conversations or games). *This was a nightly occurrence at our dinner table!*

Often, parents, teachers, or others may suspect that a child has ADHD or another attention-related disorder, but don't know when or how to seek testing. It may be difficult to tell if the behavior is typical of children that age, or if it is indeed different and concerning.

~~~~~~~~~~~~

How do I know if I should get my child tested? *A Mother's Perspective*

When my son was 7 years old, we had major changes in our family. His Grammy, who had been his primary caregiver since birth when mom and dad were at work, passed away from cancer with him in the room. A few months after that, job changes moved our family from California to Virginia, so Austin had to leave his dogs, friends, cousins, aunts and uncles, grandparents, and other extended family at home in California and move to an entirely new school and town. For the first time in his life, he no longer shared a bedroom with his older brother.

The new school classes, teachers, and schedule were overwhelming to him, and unlike when he was in school in California, he was unable to make friends at the new school. Although he had always been an excellent student and loved school, he began crying himself to sleep at night and begging to not go to school. The teachers recognized that he was having trouble making friends, and helped him get involved in after-school clubs and sports to get to know other children at another level. We got involved in the local church and youth sports leagues, but he still did not make any friends (even though he wouldn't admit it to us). We didn't suspect ADHD or any other diseases or disorders – we thought he was just having troubles adjusting to the challenges of moving clear across the country and leaving his friends and family behind. As the months continued, his behavior became more pronounced to the point that no one could have a conversation around him since he interrupted everyone so much, and the teacher for the accelerated math class asked him not to return because he would stand up at his desk constantly rather than sitting down.

He also became impulsive, even stomping his feet at daddy when he got mad (but then immediately realizing what he had done wrong and apologizing profusely). He developed a very strong sense of right and wrong, and became a tattle-tale. Even though the teacher told him other kids wouldn't want to play with him if he continued that, his impulsiveness prevented him from avoiding blurting things out to the teacher.

Although admittedly he was young before we moved from California, Austin had always been very detailed on his school work. Once starting school in Virginia, he started rushing through his school and homework, not putting enough detail into his stories for Language Arts and not showing his work in Math. He would complete his homework in 5 minutes or less, and do it correctly, but he would forget to turn it in, even with reminders. However, he was still getting straight As because he could ace the tests even if he didn't study, he could do complicated math in his head, science "just made sense" to him, and he could read a book and then remember every detail for a test. In fact, he was so good and quick at spelling, that the teacher reported this exchange at his parent-teacher conference:

The 3rd grade class was doing a spelling test, and Mrs. B was reading the word out loud, giving the kids time to spell the word on their paper, and then reading the next word. Austin was spelling very quickly and asking for the next word. Mrs. B explained she needed to give the other children time to finish spelling the word "elephant" prior to moving on to the next word. So Austin said out loud "e-l-e-p-h-a-n-t. Ok, we're all ready for the next word." The teacher thought it was really funny, and loved the fact that he spelled the word correctly, but she had to disallow him from doing it again.

His impulsiveness drove him to want to do things quickly, and if other kids were slowing him down, he would just help them whether or not they wanted the help or whether it was appropriate. He was well-known for helping other children finish their classwork or in-class projects with the hopes they would all get released for recess early. He found it very challenging to work in groups for projects, because he wanted everyone to work at his fast speed and wasn't accepting of others' ideas.

Test days were difficult, because Austin would finish the tests so quickly and have an inability to sit still and quiet while the other kids finished. Eventually, the teachers allowed him to leave the classroom and go to the library to read until the rest of the class finished the test. By the time he left elementary school, he had read every book in their library!

We were convinced to seek outside testing when his fourth grade teacher told us that she thought Austin was having anxiety attacks, because he would rapidly blink his eyes in a repetitive motion, especially when confronted with a stressful situation such as another child challenging his authority in a group setting or when the teacher requested that he sit still during a school lesson. On the way home from school that day, my son looked at my husband and said "Dad, I need help." We called that day to get him scheduled for testing.

~~~~~~~~~~~

How do I know if a child should get tested? *A Teacher's Perspective*

Many teachers are not formally trained on ADHD, nor are they trained on how to treat it. The U.S. Department of Education provided guidance for teachers on ADHD in 2003[3], but did not include any information related to nutrition and ADHD. Therefore, many will not know when it is time for a child to get tested for ADHD or be aware of any recommended nutrition interventions. School districts often will not pay for testing for behavioral problems unless the behavior is seriously adversely impacting the child's grades or other children around them. Here are some stories from my teacher friends:

Teacher 1

"Over the years I've had many students with ADHD, both already diagnosed, and some not yet. While there are many similarities from one child to the next in how they 'appear' in the classroom, there are also many differences. One word that seems to apply a lot, and fits many different categories, is SPACE. They often don't understand the unspoken boundaries of personal space. Many times they are tattled on by neighboring students who complain of them invading their space. Also, they tend to require more than average amounts of space to house their belongings. I've had the best success with ADHD students when I had the ability to seat them on an edge, or next to an empty desk on one side for all of their 'spillover' (pencils, papers, crayons, arms, head, etc.) Another aspect of space is that they have extreme difficulty confining their writing to conventional spacing on paper. Letters often fill and fall below or above the allotted space. Space between words is also not adhered to. Reading their writing is almost always a challenge. In fact, most fine motor skills are well below the average student. Another spacing issue that I've had success with is what space in the classroom best suits their needs. While the first instinct seems to be to put them in the front nearest the teacher, I've had better luck placing them in the back. When they need to stand, rather than sit, they can without affecting those behind them. They are able to take in the whole room from the back without having to turn around and therefore create a distraction for others. If they need to get up and walk it can be done with much less interruption to the rest of the class. Multiple section binders are often in the possession of my ADHD students because their parents seem to think that all they need to keep track of their work is a good organizational system. Wrong!!! I always recommend just a single folder. One side marked DONE and the other marked NOT DONE. This single folder idea is hard to grasp for the non ADHD mind, but I tell parents to trust me on this!! On the playground, they will play with anyone and everyone, but often I see that they don't have a tight group of close friends."

Teacher 2

"What I wish I could tell parents who are reluctant to get their child tested is that an ADHD diagnosis is in no way a reflection of parenting any more than a diagnosis of the common cold is! All it does is help everyone who works with their child know that there are different strategies that should be tried, and more patience to be offered. It also doesn't mean that medication is the only option. We understand that choosing to medicate a child comes with huge ramifications, but so does not properly diagnosing."

~~~~~~~~~~~

Many parents bring their child to the doctor with specific concerns about the child's ability to sustain attention, curb activity level (stay still when expected), and/or stop being impulsive. In these cases, it is clear that the doctor should initiate an evaluation for ADHD as the hallmark symptoms of ADHD are inattention, hyperactivity, and impulsivity. However, in many instances, the chief concern might include behaviors and characteristics associated with ADHD without mention of the core ADHD symptoms. These might be difficulty remaining organized, planning activities, following through with directions, or controlling their responses in certain situations. Moreover, children might have difficulty making or keeping friends, following the rules of the classroom, or regulating their behavior, mostly because of the impulsivity.

Etiology

There are a lot of big words I can (and will) use to describe the cause of ADHD, but the main point I want to make here is that ADHD isn't just "kids who move too much". There is a disruption in the regulation, or you could say disrupted communication, in the brain[1,4-6], so it is a real disease. ADHD is something that needs to be treated and managed just like any other disease would need to be. Often, just knowing that, and knowing the diagnosis, helps the child and family to cope with the symptoms much better. The irregular brain communication also explains the high rates of co-morbidities (co-occurrence) with diseases like dyslexia, depression, anxiety, and other behavioral disorders, as these all relate back to similar irregularities in the brain.

Neurotransmitters are chemicals in the brain that help the brain communicate from one neuron (brain cell) to another. These neurotransmitters are released from one neuron, travel through the synaptic space (the space between the neurons), and connect to receptors or transporters on the next neuron. These neurotransmitters need to be in this synaptic space for a certain amount of time to create the desired effect. The two neurotransmitters that are relevant to our discussion here are dopamine and serotonin.

A widely accepted theory is that children with ADHD have reduced dopamine activity in the brain, as the transporters take up too much dopamine, leaving less dopamine floating free in the synaptic space between the neurons[5]. This results in too little dopamine to control the behaviors that are associated with ADHD. People with ADHD and similar disorders also have decreased serotonin activity, which is another neurotransmitter that regulates brain activity to manage **executive function** and **sensory gating**. Executive function activities include the ability to:

- ✓ remain organized
- ✓ plan activities and think ahead
- ✓ follow through with directions
- ✓ avoid impulsive actions.

For people with reduced serotonin activity, such as those with ADHD, it is hard to manage these functions in their brain. Losing track of calculators, notebooks and assignment sheets can make it hard to complete assignments and homework. Losing track of one's own thought process can make it hard to finish essays and other executive function level tasks. The child may struggle with breaking down a school assignment or a household job into steps and getting started, or planning ahead to determine what he should do next. It also is very difficult to control impulsive actions, such as interrupting or tattle-telling, when the executive functioning centers of the brain are not working correctly.

Additionally, people with ADHD have a reduced ability for sensory gating (also known as filtering). This describes the neurological process of filtering out unnecessary stimuli and preventing an overload of irrelevant information in the higher cortical centers of the brain. For most of us, we can sit in a classroom or movie theater or at the dinner table and concentrate on the task at hand despite multiple other things happening all around us. Someone tapping their feet, butterflies outside the window, another kid sharpening a pencil, or someone else humming a tune are things that most children can filter out to focus on the task at hand such as the school lesson being taught. But for a child with ADHD who doesn't have this sensory gating function, he cannot filter it out and therefore has a harder time focusing on the lesson being taught or what he is supposed to do next. This could also explain the irritability and social behaviors that can be experienced by children with ADHD – for example, he may decide not to eat lunch with other kids at school because he gets so annoyed by the sound of others chewing (because he can't filter it out) or may skip social situations such as the movie theater due to multiple competing stimuli in that environment. I have heard from other parents and healthcare professionals that kids with ADHD get too hot or feel like they're too stuck in a tight spot at times. People with ADHD explain that lights get too bright, clothes are too irritating, and that they are unable to ignore the second -hand on their watch. All of these symptoms can lead to difficulties with behavior in social situations, which can be challenging for children who spend most of their days at school and other social settings.

Before Austin controlled his ADHD, mealtimes were very challenging for him because he could hear his brother chewing and it bothered him greatly. No one else at the table could hear him, or if we did, we were filtering it out and ignoring it. Austin would make frequent movements away from his brother, which was disruptive to the family and hurtful to Tyler. Tyler began to look for a place to sit away from his brother to avoid the interaction. As parents, we had to balance the needs of the two children to come to a compromise that worked for our family.

It's believed that a child with ADHD may have difficulty or the inability to shut down the right brain in favor of the left brain as many of us normally do. So while this can lead the child to be impulsive and inattentive, they are also usually creative, innovative, and imaginative. These children are often the builders, creators, engineers, inventors, and chefs. Because they have not mastered sensory gating or filtering out external stimuli, if they can learn to harness what are extraneous, blocked stimuli to others they can become the musical geniuses, creative thinkers, and entrepreneurs. Often, they are the super intelligent children as well.

> At the age of 2, Austin was building full Lego sets and 100+ piece puzzles. I have heard from many of the families I work with that their children with ADHD can play musical instruments better than anyone else in the family and they are fascinated with the way bridges and skyscrapers are built.

In fact, many famously successful people have discussed their ADHD diagnoses. Michael Phelps says that he used swimming as an activity to help him focus. Walt Disney was the creative genius behind an empire – but he surrounded himself by others who could work out the details to which he couldn't pay attention. Justin Timberlake has discussed his ADHD publicly, and similarly to others with ADHD he is a creative and musical genius. Michael Jordan is known as a basketball legend, but that's not all – he has his own line of shoes and several other merchandise lines. He has always looked for his next move, with creativity that he has contributed to his ADHD. Richard Branson, who is the billionaire entrepreneur who has funded the commercial space flight industry, has ADHD – to which he credits his imagination and innovation. Success stories like these will continue to help remove the negative stereotypes surrounding ADHD.

We have focused on serotonin and dopamine in this chapter, but it's important to know that when one neurotransmitter is out of balance, the metabolism, synthesis, and uptake of other neurotransmitters can be impaired.

As reduced dopamine activity in the brain is often blamed for the symptoms caused by ADHD[6], medical treatment for ADHD usually involves treatment with methylphenidate or amphetamine-containing medications. These act on the dopamine receptors to allow dopamine to stay in the spaces between the neurons longer and perform their required functions. These medications are therefore classified as stimulant medications, which seems counterintuitive in the management of a hyperactive disorder. *Why would you want to stimulate a child who is already hyperactive?* However, the stimulant action is in the brain, and is beneficial for increasing neuronal activity, not in increasing hyperactivity.

One thing that isn't often realized is that there is a genetic component to ADHD[7]! This means that if a child has ADHD, a close relative probably does too. If that other person is a parent or primary caregiver, this may make management of the disease more challenging as that person will need to learn to control their own behaviors in addition to those of their child(ren).

Prevalence

I bet some of you reading this are wondering how prevalent this disease is. If your child is in an elementary class with 30 students, how many of them are likely to have ADHD? That partially depends on how many of those students are boys, and how many are girls. As of 2011, the Centers for Disease Control and Prevention (CDC) had reported that about 11% of children have been diagnosed with ADHD[8]. Estrogen is a hormone that girls produce in much greater quantities than boys, and this helps ensure adequate serotonin levels. Therefore, about half as many girls are diagnosed with ADHD as boys (13.2% of boys were diagnosed with ADHD as opposed to 5.6% of girls according to the same 2011 CDC report). According to a study reported in *Pediatrics* in 2013[9], black and Hispanic children are less likely to be diagnosed with ADHD than white children. None of this includes, of course, the children who have ADHD but have not been formally diagnosed.

So to answer the question, the odds are that at least 4 children in that class of 30 have been formally diagnosed with ADHD, and it depends on how many are girls versus how many are boys and the ethnic composition of the class.

MORE FACTS ABOUT THE PREVALENCE OF ADHD IN THE U.S.

Average age of diagnosis:
      Mild ADHD -- 8 years old
      Moderate ADHD -- 7 years old
      Severe ADHD -- 5 years old

11% of U.S. children diagnosed with ADHD in 2011 = 6.4 million children.
      A little more than half of those children, 3.5 million, were taking medications to treat their ADHD.
      No statistics were given on how many were also using any kinds of nutritional treatments for their ADHD.

School administrators, guidance counselors, and teachers have frequently told me in several different school districts that they "don't worry about ADHD, because over half the school has it". When I hear this, I immediately know there is a lack of knowledge on the diagnosis and prevalence of ADHD. Although the 11% reported by the CDC only includes those who have been formally diagnosed and likely doesn't include all of the cases, it would be a very big jump to assume that over 50% of the school aged population has it. This concerns me, because I don't think that ADHD should be dismissed as a casual condition. Many of these same people also tell me things like "we just recommend they take a physical activity class as their elective to get the wiggles out". This proves there are still many misconceptions about ADHD and the required treatment that is much more complex than just getting 30-60 minutes of activity per day! (Check out the exercise chapter for more on this issue!)

So as you can see, ADHD is a brain-based disorder that can be treated. This explains why a lot of children with ADHD are diagnosed with other behavioral disorders, as there are similar etiologies (causes) for these disorders. The table illustrates the percent of children with ADHD who also have these other disorders.

2007 National Survey of Children's Health (based on parent reports)
- Learning disabilities -- 46%
- Conduct disorder -- 27%
- Anxiety -- 18%
- Depression -- 14%
- Speech problems -- 12%

Doctors refer to the presence of other diseases that are present at the same time as "comorbidities". Some conditions have similar symptoms as ADHD, which is why a full evaluation is required to be sure the child's issues are properly identified and an appropriate treatment program is started. Here are some issues that often coexist with ADHD[10,11]:

- **Learning disabilities.** Some learning disabilities make it hard for children to stay organized. Children with certain forms of dyslexia have trouble processing and responding to directions (written or spoken).

- **Behavior disorders- Oppositional Defiant Disorder (ODD) and Conduct Disorder (CD).** These two disorders can be the most challenging co-morbidities of ADHD (and they can occur independently of ADHD). Children with these disorders often are very aggressive and disruptive. A child diagnosed with ADHD who is having extreme behavior difficulties should probably be further evaluated for ODD and/or CD.

- **Emotional regulation issues.** This includes mental health conditions such as anxiety disorders, depression, and obsessive-compulsive disorders that can cause symptoms beyond a child's control. These are more than just temporary emotional difficulties that all children have. Some of those symptoms are also seen with ADHD, such as emotional outbursts, high energy and the need to have things happen in a certain way.

- **Social (pragmatic) communication disorder.** This condition makes it hard for a child to engage in socially appropriate conversations. Kids with this disorder may easily become irritable due to trouble understanding body language, puns, sarcasm and statements that don't mean exactly what they say.

- **Auditory processing disorder.** This can make it hard for kids to understand and follow spoken directions. There's a disconnect between the ear and brain, making a child appear inattentive or unable to follow directions. A child may have both auditory processing disorder and ADHD, but sometimes one gets misdiagnosed for the other.

- **Motor and oral (vocal) tic disorders.** Although the most commonly known tic disorder is Tourette syndrome, there are others as well. Tic disorders can cause body movements and vocal sounds that kids can't control.

We first sought out a diagnosis for Austin because of his tic disorder. He would make very soft noises as though he was constantly clearing his throat and his eyes would flutter rapidly, and he wasn't aware that he was doing this. We noticed that this tended to occur more often in stressful situations, such as whenever we would ask him about school or an assignment, or when he would go to a new social situation. His teacher reported that it happened often at school, especially when she spoke directly to him. We thought it was indicative of anxiety disorder, but found out when we got his final diagnoses that tic disorders are conditions in and of themselves and are often associated with ADHD.

ADHD and many of the issues described above share a common thread: the executive functioning issues that we discussed already. Executive functioning skills allow us to plan, organize, remember things, pay attention and get started on tasks. A child with ADHD or another disorder may not be able to do these executive functions, making daily activities more challenging.

We have talked a lot in this chapter about the signs and symptoms that might suggest a child has ADHD, and we have discussed the physiological causes for ADHD in the brain. We have focused on the hallmark characteristics of ADHD: inattention, hyperactivity, and impulsivity. Now, I want to share some stories that children with ADHD have told me to help me understand what it's actually like to live with ADHD.

Living with ADHD
Video games

Although Austin had a PS3 gaming system, he rarely used it and much preferred using my iPhone for simple app games. Later, we learned that many children with ADHD and other similar brain-based diseases do not like video games! Have you ever read the warnings on the back of a video game? Most of them say *"A very small percentage of individuals may experience epileptic seizures when exposed to certain light patterns or flashing lights. Exposure to certain light patterns or backgrounds on a television screen or while playing video games may induce an epileptic seizure in these individuals…If you experience e any of the following symptoms while playing a video game – dizziness, altered vision, eye or muscle twitches, low of awareness, disorientation, any involuntary movement, or convulsions – contact your physician immediately."* It is thought that for some people who have trouble filtering out extraneous stimuli, like children with ADHD, the frames per second of many video games is too overwhelming for these children on a subconscious level so they avoid them without even knowing why. This certainly explained for us why Austin preferred iPhone apps more than video games!

Note: While I have met several other children with ADHD who are similar to my son in avoiding fast-paced video games, other children with ADHD prefer fast moving video games rather than slower app type games, which can be attributed to the hallmark traits of ADHD of impulsivity and inattentiveness. While it may seem that the child is paying more attention for a longer period of time to video games than school work, it really is due to the fact that video games actually require short bursts of attention to different tasks and fast responses with immediate gratification (such as the player living or dying, or the points earned or lost, or whatever the response of the game is).

Many children with ADHD don't read full novels, or read much at all, because of their inattentiveness and restlessness. However, Austin loves to read because of his strong imagination and ability to immerse himself in the setting and identify with the characters in a book.

Field Trips

Austin's class had a field trip to the Art Museum at the University of Virginia (UVA), and to tour the Rotunda designed by Thomas Jefferson that hosted the first classes at UVA. I chaperoned the trip, so I could spend time with my son, learn more about the history of the area, and monitor his behavior. The day was exhausting for me, because Austin was constantly either whispering to me or moving excessively or staring out the window or interrupting the tour guide with (what seemed like) random questions. I came home with the impression that the field trip was a waste of time for Austin. However, at dinner that night telling his dad and older brother about the day, he recounted almost every word that the tour guide had said and every detail of the rooms we toured! Later I learned that it is actually helpful for children with ADHD to move when they're learning. It is theorized that the movement enhances brain activity, and this may be true even for children without ADHD. This experience taught me that even if my son didn't appear to be listening, he was soaking in much more than I thought.

I look forward to the day when people no longer make assumptions that people with ADHD are trouble makers or not intelligent. When children with ADHD hear of so many amazingly successful people having the same disease as them, it gives them hope for their own future. I believe there is less of a stigma these days about having ADHD, but we do still have work to do to educate people. Thankfully, people are realizing that they can say "Wow, you're so lucky that your child has ADHD!"

When my son started middle school, he didn't mind going to the nurse during the day. In fact, he went at the same time as 2 other kids in his class with ADHD to get their medication, and they all discussed their dosages and the names of the medications they were on, what it felt like to have ADHD, what their friends thought about it, and other things about ADHD while they walked to the nurses office together. It was like they had formed their own support group!

Chapter 2 References
1. American Psychiatric Association: Diagnostic and Statistical Manual of Mental Disorders, Fifth Edition.
Arlington, VA, American Psychiatric Association, 2013.

2. DSM-5TM. ADHD Institute website. Available at http://www.adhd-institute.com/assessment-diagnosis/diagnosis/dsm-5tm/. Updated February 2017. Accessed March 27, 2017.

3. ADHD Identifying and treating Attention Deficit Hyperactivity Disorder: A resource for school and home, 2003. U.S. Department of Education website. Available at https://www2.ed.gov/teachers/needs/speced/adhd/adhd-

resource-pt1.pdf. Updated August 2003.Accessed March 27, 2017.

4. Volkow ND, Wang GJ, Newcorn J, et al. Brain dopamine transporter levels in treatment and drug naive adults with ADHD. *Neuroimage* 2007;34:1182–1190.

5. Banaschewski T, Hollis C, Oosterlaan J, Roeyers H, Rubia K, Willcutt E. Towards an understanding of unique and shared pathways in the psychopathophysiology of ADHD. *Dev. Sci.* 2005;8; 132–140.

6. Dopamine and ADHD. DNA Learning Center website. Available at https://www.dnalc.org/view/841-Dopamine-and-ADHD.html. Accessed March 27, 2017.

7. Biederman J, Spencer T. Attention-deficit/hyperactivity disorder (ADHD) as a noradrenergic disorder. *Biol Psychiatry*. 1999;46:1234-1242.

8. Key Findings: Trends in the Parent-Report of Health Care Provider Diagnosed and Medicated ADHD: United States, 2003—2011. Centers for Disease Control and Prevention website. Available at https://www.cdc.gov/ncbddd/adhd/features/key-findings-adhd72013.html. Updated December 10, 2014. Accessed March 27, 2017.

9. Morgan PL, Staff J, Hillemeier MM, Farkas G, Maczuga S., Racial and ethnic disparities in ADHD diagnosis from kindergarten to eighth grade, *Pediatrics*. 2013;132:85-93.

10. Spencer TJ, Biederman J, Mick E. Attention-deficit/hyperactivity disorder: diagnosis, lifespan, comorbidities, and neurobiology. *Ambul Pediatr.* 2007;7:73-81.

11. Connor DF, Edwards G, Fletcher KE, Baird J, Barkley RA, Steingard RJ. Correlates of comorbid psychopathology in children with ADHD. *J Am Acad Child Adolesc Psychiatry*. 2003;42:193-200.

3 LAWS RELATED TO SERVICES FOR CHILDREN WITH ADHD IN PUBLIC SCHOOLS

This chapter is included in a book about nutrition management strategies for children with ADHD because a major influencer on children's' lives and food environment is the school setting. I included a table on the laws that are specifically related to the rights of ADHD students to a free, appropriate public education (FAPE) in the United States. Since children spend a large amount of time in school, parents and caregivers need to be empowered to advocate for their children when needed. Understanding the laws and "speaking the language" of the school administrators will be very valuable for this.

LAWS RELATED TO SERVICES FOR CHILDREN WITH ADHD IN PUBLIC SCHOOLS	
Americans with Disabilities Act, Amendments Act of 2008[1] (known as the Amendments Act)	Broadened the interpretation of terms that define disability in two ways of particular significance for students with ADHD. • Expanded the list of examples of major life activities by adding concentrating, reading, thinking, and functions of the brain. • Stated that mitigating measures shall not be considered in determining whether an individual has a disability.

	○ Mitigating measures for ADHD include medications, coping strategies, and adaptive neurological modifications that an individual could use to eliminate or reduce the effects of an impairment. ○ The impact of a student's ADHD on a given major life activity, such as concentrating or thinking, must be considered in the student's untreated state to determine whether a substantial limitation exists. For example, if a student requires medication to control the ADHD, the child's behaviors or disabilities without the medication are the ones considered when evaluating the student for a disability.
Section 504 of the Rehabilitation Act of 1973[2] (usually referred to simply as "Section 504")	▪ Administered by the United States Department of Education, Office for Civil Rights (OCR) ▪ Prohibits discrimination on the basis of disability in programs or activities receiving Federal financial assistance, including schools. ▪ Requires Free Appropriate Public Education (FAPE) with accommodations to address the disability on an individual basis. ▪ The definition of disability is the same under both Title II and Section 504. Under these laws, a student with

	a disability is one who has a physical or mental impairment that substantially limits one or more major life activities. **Some examples of a major life activity that could be substantially limited by ADHD include concentrating, reading, thinking, and functions of the brain.**
Individuals with Disabilities Education Act (IDEA)[3]	▪ Requires States and school districts to ensure students with disabilities receive appropriate special education and related services at no cost to the parents (FAPE) ▪ This is the primary method for identifying, evaluating, and educating students with disabilities who need special education and related services.

In summary, the Amendments Act of the Americans with Disability Act clarified that ADHD could legally be considered a protected disability. Section 504 requires that all Americans with a disability receive a free education that is appropriate to their individual needs. Often, schools will refer to setting up a 504 plan for the child. The IDEA requires the FAPE as well, and is the primary method for identifying children who need special services and providing education with necessary accommodations.

According to the Office of Civil Rights (OCR)[2], who administers Section 504, many teachers are not familiar with ADHD, or how it could impact a student's equal access to a school district's program. After receiving 2,000 complaints of discrimination against students with ADHD from 2011-2015, they created a guidance document for school districts in July 2016. This resource guide is in the public domain, meaning it is accessible and reproducible by anyone who needs it. This guide is also available on the OCR's website at http://www.ed.gov/ocr; U.S. Department of Education, Office for Civil Rights, *Students with ADHD and Section 504: A Resource Guide* (July 2016).

School districts must conduct *individualized* evaluations of students who, because of disability, including ADHD, need or are believed to need special education or related services, and must ensure that qualified students with disabilities receive appropriate services that are based on specific needs, not cost, and not based on stereotypes or generalized misunderstanding of a disability.

I emphasize the word *individualized* because of my experience working with school administrators, teachers, and other school district staff on behalf of my own son or other children. There are many misconceptions about ADHD and their responsibilities for helping these children in the school setting. I commonly hear them say "we don't do anything special for children with ADHD because over half our school has ADHD", Since only 11% of children actually are diagnosed with ADHD using validated methods, it just isn't possible to have over half the school with ADHD unless no other school in the district has more than a handful of children with ADHD. They often further qualify it with "we have a lot of boys in this school, that's why we have so much ADHD", which again can't be true. The 2013 CDC report stated that 13.2% of boys were diagnosed with ADHD (compared to5.6% of girls), so it is true that classes with more boys than girls are more likely to have more ADHD than classes with more girls. However, it is still pretty close to impossible to have "more than half of the school" with ADHD.

Even if that were true, the laws make it clear that they need to individually evaluate every child with any disability, including ADHD, to ensure a free, *appropriate* public education. Assuming that every child with ADHD has the same educational and environmental needs is erroneous and discriminatory and harmful. School districts cannot simply group together a few services and provide them in a general fashion to any student with ADHD. Many of these same teachers or school officials will also say, "we just encourage them to take P.E. electives so they can get the wiggles out", which further shows that they do not understand ADHD or the individual needs of their students. ADHD is NOT "the wiggles". Running and playing and jumping will NOT cure ADHD (see chapter 6 for a discussion on exercise's effects on ADHD). Certainly, ignorance or a dismissive attitude on behalf of people who run our children's schools, where they spend so much of their time, will not help the problem of misconception and misunderstanding of these children or the disease.

Please know, I am not trying to be critical of teachers or school administrators. My children have had many amazing teachers and coaches, and I have many friends and family members who are teachers. They have had a positive influence in my family's lives. Many of my friends and family members who are teachers will be the first to tell me they have not learned enough about ADHD symptoms, etiology, or treatment and are looking forward to learning more so that they can help their students. Since there are many school officials and teachers who carry these misconceptions, probably unintentionally, it is our jobs as health professionals and parents to advocate for our children by educating the school districts.

If I had the chance to speak to all teachers, I would tell them this:

ADHD is a brain based disease, with abnormalities in the neurotransmitters in the brain. It causes impulsivity, inattention, and hyperactivity with varying degrees of severity. Some children are not hyperactive but are impulsive and inattentive, or could display any combination of these symptoms. Many of them are geniuses, and therefore have learned to overcome their disease so that you don't recognize that they have it. A child who is doing well academically still may be struggling to reach their full potential.

Consider the fact that the kid who finishes an hour's worth of work in 10 minutes maybe isn't skimping on the work or being lazy. Perhaps he is a genius, and he doesn't need an hour to do it, and he's really bored for the other 50 minutes of class. When he's talking to the kid sitting next to him, check to see what they're talking about rather than automatically getting him in trouble. It's very possible that he's teaching the other kid how to do the math, because he can translate what you're saying into something his friend understands. Instead of demoting him to a lower level math class for talking, perhaps it would be better to engage him more fully in the current class or move him to a higher level class to put that genius math brain to better use.

Chapter 5 shares tips for crafting the school environment to improve nutrition intake and mealtime behaviors for children with ADHD.

Chapter 3 References

1. ADA Amendments Act of 2008. U.S. Equal Employment Opportunity Commission website. Available at https://www.eeoc.gov/laws/statutes/adaaa.cfm. Updated September 25, 2008. Accessed March 27, 2017.

2. Dear colleague letter and resource guide on students with ADHD. United States Department of Education Office for Civil Rights. July 26, 2016.

3. Individuals with Disabilities Education Act (IDEA 2004). U.S. Department of Education website. Available at http://idea.ed.gov/. Updated February 16, 2017. Accessed March 27, 2017.

I mentioned that we had my son tested to determine what was causing his impulsivity, nervous tics, and inattention. The psychologist told us that he is a genius with ADHD. When we asked for strategies to help him remember to turn in his homework, his response really helped put things in perspective for us. He told us to work with his teachers to "Get a system in place to help him turn in his homework, even if it meant a personal reminder from the teacher each day or twice an hour". He said "his brilliant mind needed to concentrate on more important things, like curing cancer". While we *certainly* understand and promote the importance and value of completing routine, every-day tasks like turning in his homework and following through on assignments and learning to work in a group, it did help us to see the bigger picture and stop fighting little battles. Some teachers were more willing to help him with those details than others, but consistently each year we set up a system at home with positive feedback when he does complete routine tasks like turning in his homework every day for a week. This is an example of when I say that sometimes just having a diagnosis and a recognition that ADHD is a real disease can make a big difference in a family's ability to deal with the disease.

4 NUTRITION RESEARCH FOR ADHD

When Austin was diagnosed with ADHD, we honestly had no real idea what that meant. Although we had heard the term a lot and had heard that children with ADHD moved a lot, we didn't know any of the real details. We checked out books from the library for my husband and I to understand the brain-based etiology of the disease, and we checked out books that were more appropriate for Austin to learn about his disease at a 10 year old level. We researched ADHD treatments and what we could do to help our son, which included medications and family based behavior therapy. Each night, Austin would sit with me to read one chapter in the books we had checked out. My husband and I would have conversations with him about how the medications made him feel, what he thought about the disease, what questions he had, what he was learning from the books, and detailed questions about his school work. We set up a positive reward system for small "wins" at school or home, like not interrupting at mealtime and turning in his homework every day. We met with his teachers and came up with a plan for them to gently give Austin a personal reminder if he didn't put his work in the in-basket or to quietly excuse him to the library to read a book if he finished his test early. We worked with the psychologist in a ten week family behavior therapy program to learn how to craft the home environment to help Austin be successful.

As a registered dietitian, I was also curious if there were any nutrition interventions that had been proven to help children with ADHD or other disorders that shared the hallmark characteristics of inattention, hyperactivity, and impulsivity. For the first time ever, I went on parenting and nutrition blogs to see what others were doing for their children with ADHD. I was dismayed (although I shouldn't have been surprised) by the sensational information that is "published" on these blogs, with a complete lack of scientific evidence for what is being recommended. Many of the writers were very persuasive, and other parents seemed to be trying very hard to follow their advice even at a high monetary and peace-of-mind cost to themselves and their families. It is hard enough to have a child with ADHD, then to try medications to figure out which ones work without horrible side effects and work with teachers for a school 504 plan and change routines at home and educate siblings and friends and yourselves and help the child understand his diagnosis and cope with the fact that he might be taking medication for the rest of his life and tell you he feels like *"all we ever do as a family anymore is talk about his disease"* and .... you get the point! I only wanted to do nutrition interventions that had at least been proven to work.

I decided to do a literature review of primary research done in the area of nutrition and ADHD to find out the real evidence for myself; as I read through all of this complicated material I decided I needed to educate others with what I learned. This book is one of the ways I am sharing with parents, caregivers, teachers, children, and other healthcare professionals what I have learned by reading this research, along with practical tips from using these strategies with my own son and other children who have been diagnosed with ADHD. For the benefit of the dietitians and other healthcare professionals reading this book, I will share statistics and scientific information about the studies; for those of you who are reading this to learn more about what to do for your own children or someone you care about, I will translate that into practical every day tips that you can use.

Conducting research studies for ADHD

Before we go any further into the results of scientific studies on nutrition and ADHD, it is important to discuss how these studies are completed. The anthropometric and some of the other studies that we will discuss are based on objective data, or data that is quantifiable (able to be put into numbers) and directly measurable. Most of the rest of the studies are based on subjective data, which is qualitative information from a person's point of view (their perception of what did or didn't happen). Although there is no standardized questionnaire suitable for the purpose of this type of study, parental report of behavior in ADHD children is considered to be the most reliable source of information for this patient population[1]. There are different validated tools used by psychologists and psychiatrists to test for behavior based disorders including ADHD, with none of them being recognized as the gold standards against which to compare the others. Sometimes more than one of these questionnaire-type tools will be used to determine the appropriate diagnosis, such as in the comprehensive testing that we got for our son. In those cases, many of the questions are repeated from one questionnaire to the next, and it can be tiresome for the parents or teachers to complete them all. We answered hundreds of questions about our son both at the beginning of the 8 week testing period and at the end.

Since testing is often done at the primary care or family medicine physician's office, where they have less time to dig deeper into the behavior details and usually don't have the equipment to measure actual movements (such as the actigraphs used in the research study for my son), only one questionnaire is used. If the responses indicate a score that meets a certain threshold, then the child is diagnosed with ADHD, without a deeper investigation or diagnosis process. I have also heard from parents that they told the doctor they thought their child had ADHD and they were therefore given the diagnosis and medication. I think this is why teachers and school administrators will say "half of our school has ADHD", because the diagnosis methods are so varied.

Often, published research studying an intervention with children diagnosed with ADHD do not distinguish the testing method that was used to determine if the child does in fact have ADHD. At some extent though, one has to trust that the children who are subjects in these studies do, in fact, have ADHD and not some other disorder or behavior problem. A more significant challenge with conducting these studies is what is known as the Hawthorne effect – where people behave differently when they know they're being watched[2]. These studies almost always involve parent (and sometimes teacher or other caregiver) *perception* of behavior as the outcome measurements are the parents' and/or teachers' answers on the same questionnaire before and after the intervention period. When a parent learns that their child has a disease, he/she usually want to DO something to help their child, and the act of doing something (anything) during an intervention period they think is helping is highly likely to change their perception of their child's behavior and therefore their answers on a questionnaire.

We also have to consider the ethics of studies conducted on children, which is why there is sometimes a limited sample size or few studies conducted. To be truly designed well, a study would have three groups: children who have not been diagnosed with ADHD, children who have been diagnosed with ADHD but are not taking medications to treat it, and children who have been diagnosed with ADHD and are taking medications to treat it. This can help researchers understand if the intervention is effective on children with ADHD simply because it is effective on all children, and it can help understand if the treatment effect is independent of medication treatment or rather is an additive effect to the improvement seen with medication therapy. Larger sample sizes can help reduce the possibility of random chance error. It is very difficult, however, to get participation from large numbers of children from each of these groups to participate in these studies. Many also consider it unethical to withhold treatment that could be beneficial for a child simply for the sake of research, or to possibly subject a child to an intervention that hasn't proven to be 100% safe already. There is also tremendous costs associated with these studies, which can be a limitation when funding sources are limited.

This book will share a lot of information about nutrition studies! But reading the original research is not how most people learn about ADHD. Adding to the difficulty of conducting studies in the first place, most people learn their "research" about nutrition and ADHD through the media. Rarely do people have access to and read the original research studies (such as the ones I discuss in this book), and many are difficult to understand by the general public anyway. Even when the media does refer to primary research that was conducted, often they are putting a media-worthy slant on it or using it to promote products they are selling.

For example, by reading this website pictured here, the internet reader might think that "an influential study" showed that food dyes increase hyperactivity. They may then think their child may be hyperactive (without even knowing a true definition of hyperactivity) not because of a misconnection in the brain neurotransmitters but because of intake of artificial food colors. They might then work very hard to omit all foods with these substances and not seek medical help for a disease or seek nutrition advice to ensure adequate growth. When reading further on the internet page, it does say that "it should be noted that the FDA reports that studies have not yet proven a connection between synthetic additives in hyperactivity." Unfortunately, many don't read past the headlines. The picture below it is the actual article that is referenced by the website[3]. The original study was completed on 3 year olds, and they weren't even diagnosed with ADHD. Furthermore, the only evaluation metric was parent perception of the behavior of their 3 year old children. The article referenced on this website meant to help parents of children with ADHD isn't even a study about children with ADHD!

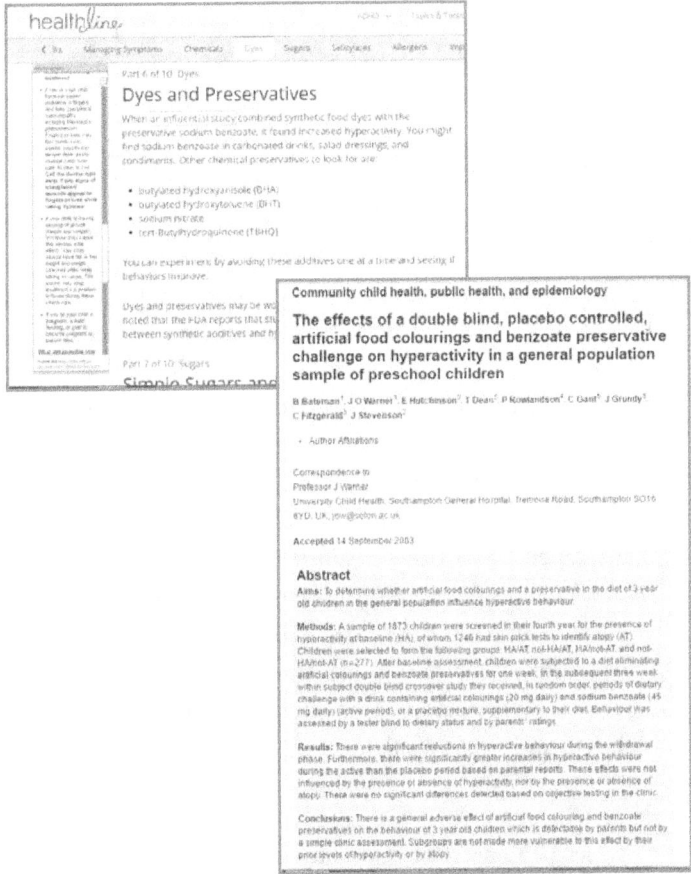

As healthcare professionals, it is our responsibility to evaluate the primary source literature and help parents and children interpret the relevance of the findings to their own situation. This involves an evaluation of sample size, intervention methods, control and intervention groups, evaluation criteria (i.e. objective vs subjective data), diagnosis criteria, and several other factors. Parents and caregivers should also do their best to evaluate these factors and seek out help from a trusted medical professional and/or registered dietitian if needed.

The American Academy of Pediatrics published guidelines for ADHD management in 2011 from their Task Force on Mental Health[4], and while medication and behavioral therapy were included nutrition therapy was not. The American Academy of Children and Adolescent Psychiatry also does not address nutritional treatments for ADHD[5]. Although nutritional interventions are not necessarily the first thing many people consider to treat ADHD, the increase in online support groups and blog posts regarding the subject seem to be increasing attention on possible nutritional influences on ADHD management.[6,7] I believe (and hope) that with recent research focusing on nutrition management that future versions of these guidelines will include a nutritional component. With that background, let's start reviewing some of the research, its practical implications for our children, and strategies that have been proven to work!

Chapter 4 References

1. Russell G, Rodgers LR, Ukoumunne OC, Ford T. Prevalence of parent-reported ASD and ADHD in the
UK: Findings from the Millennium Cohort Study. *J Autism Dev Disord.* 2014;44(1):31–34.

2. McCambridge J, Witton J, Elbourne DR. Systematic review of the Hawthorne effect: New concepts are needed to study research participation effects. *J Clin Epidemiol.* 2014;67:267-277.

3. Bateman B, Warner JO, Hutchinson E, et al. The effects of a double blind, placebo controlled, artificial food colourings and benzoate preservative challenge on hyperactivity in a general population sample of preschool children. *Arch Dis Child.* 2004;89:506-511.

4. ADHD: Clinical practice guideline for the diagnosis, evaluation, and treatment of ADHD in children and adolescents. *Pediatrics.* 2011;128:1-16.

5. Practice parameter for the assessment and treatment of children and adolescents with ADHD. *J. Am. Acad. Child Adolesc. Psychiatry.* 2007;46:894-921.

6. The best ADHD blogs of the year. Healthline Web site. http://www.healthline.com/healthslideshow/ best-adhd-blogs. Updated April 23, 2014. Accessed July 2, 2014.

7. Healthy Bites: ADHD and Diet. Brain Balance Achievement Center Web site. http://www.brainbalancecenters.com/blog/2013/01/healthy-bites-adhd-and-diet/. Updated January 2013. Accessed July 2, 2014.

5 NUTRITION CONSIDERATIONS

Eating Behaviors of Children with ADHD

To develop recommended nutrition interventions for ADHD, we need to understand the typical eating behaviors of these children. In 2014, Ptacek et al[1] investigated eating behaviors and lifestyle factors that may explain the increased incidence of obesity in children diagnosed with ADHD prior to receiving adequate treatment. Eating habits were assessed from structured interviews of parents of boys aged 6 to 10 years old, comparing 100 boys diagnosed with ADHD to 100 boys of the same age without ADHD. None of the children were taking medications for treatment of ADHD symptoms. This research demonstrated that ADHD children frequently skip meals more often than the other children, yet they eat more than five times per day in a pattern commonly known as "grazing"[1]. Therefore, they eat on a less defined schedule but more frequently. Children with ADHD also drink more sugar sweetened beverages (SSBs) than the other children, accounting for almost half of daily fluid intake (this means they don't drink very much water or non-caloric beverages). Parents of ADHD children were less likely to report that their children ate fruits and vegetables than parents of children without ADHD. Further worsening the problem is the fact that ADHD children spent more hours watching television or playing on a computer than children in the non-ADHD group. Children in the non-ADHD group spent on average two hours more per day in sports activities.

Other researchers have produced similar results to Ptacek's findings, confirming lower self-control in eating[2,3] and poor meal planning with the tendency to eat what is convenient and readily available[4]. Banaschewski et al[5] demonstrated that ADHD children choose the immediate choice when faced with immediate food choices versus delayed food choices. Often, the immediate choices are not the healthy choices.

Anthropometrics

"Anthropometrics" means body measurements – which includes height, weight, head circumference, mid-arm circumference, and lots of other measurements. A person's anthropometric measurements are then compared against reference standards. Children are compared using standardized growth charts; several are available, with the most commonly used ones published by the Centers for Disease Control and Prevention (CDC). These growth charts use actual measurements of thousands of children in the United States of a given age and gender, and establish average percentiles. For example, a child at the 50th percentile height for age is estimated to be taller than half of children his age and shorter than the other half. Plotting a child's anthropometric measurements over time on a growth chart can indicate if he is growing at the rate expected for his age. The growth charts and further explanations on their development can be found on the CDC's website at www.cdc.gov/growthcharts.

BMI	Weight Status
18.4 and lower	Underweight
18.5 to 24.9	Normal weight
25 – 29.9	Overweight
30+	Obese

Growth charts are not the only way that a child should be monitored for nutritional status and health, but they are helpful for forming an overall understanding of their health and nutrition status. Body mass index (BMI) is a measurement that compares a person's weight with their height, using the equation of {height in meters divided by weight kilograms squared} or {m/kg²}. Weight status as indicated by BMI for adults is explained in the table. Comparison of their BMI against the average standard using the CDC growth charts can explain the weight status of a child. A child is considered underweight if their body mass index (BMI) for age is less than the 5th percentile. He is considered overweight if the BMI for age is greater than the 85th but less than the 95th percentile, and obese if greater than the 95th percentile BMI/age. Short stature is defined as less than the 3rd percentile height for age. However, serial measurements plotted over time to monitor the trend of the growth is considered to be more important than the actual point on the chart. A snapshot of one of the growth charts is included on the next page, but the CDC website should be used to obtain charts for plotting growth if needed.

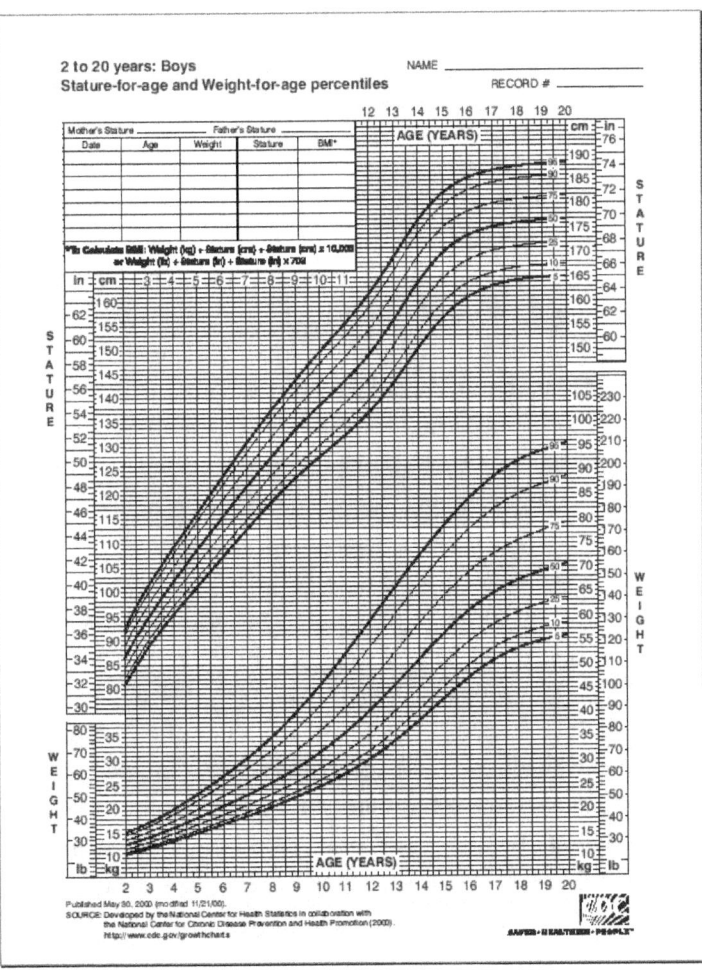

EFFECT OF ADHD ON HEIGHT

By 2005, 29 research papers had been published reporting the trends in growth in height of children using stimulant medications to treat ADHD[6]. Since some of these reports provided inconsistent results, a physician named Dr. Poulton evaluated all 29 of these studies. His conclusion was that studies that were designed well with reliable methods all consistently showed a slower rate of growth in height of approximately 1 cm per year for the first 3 years of medication treatment. This means that children grew about one inch less than expected during the first 3 years of taking stimulant medications (2.54 cm = 1 inch). There was limited data that rebound growth may be possible if medication use is stopped, meaning that some of the children caught back up on the missed growth once they stopped taking the medication. In 2009, another researcher[7] used more complex anthropometric measurements to investigate whether the slower growth was more strongly related to medication treatment of ADHD, or to the disease itself. Fifty-two boys with ADHD not treated with medication and 52 boys with ADHD treated with the stimulant medication methylphenidate (aka Ritalin) were compared to the population norm (i.e. the CDC growth charts). Findings suggested that the decreased rate of growth for height may be related to the disease itself, not the treatment with the stimulant medication. Further research in this area should include larger groups of children with a control group of children without ADHD to compare to children with ADHD with and without treatment of stimulant medication. In the meantime, most clinicians, parents, and children will consider the benefits of treatment with stimulant medications to outweigh the risks of the possible slightly slower growth in height. According to the earlier research as evaluated by Dr. Poulton[6], most children still achieve an acceptable adult height, but this reduction in rate of growth in height should be monitored on a regular basis and addressed if needed.

EFFECT OF ADHD ON WEIGHT

Contrary to the conventional thought that the increased movement in hyperactive children leads to the child being underweight, children with ADHD are actually more likely to be overweight or obese if they have not started on medications[8-13]. A large study called the National Survey of Children's Health, conducted in 2003-2004, included 62,887 children and adolescents aged 5 to 17 years and confirmed the earlier studies on obesity and ADHD[14]. This was significant because of the very large sample size. Children with ADHD not taking stimulant medications were 1.5 times more likely to be overweight.

Most authors relate the increase in overweight and obesity to a lower self-control in many lifestyle aspects, including eating-related behaviors. Impulsive children showed an increased calorie consumption when presented with foods that varied in color, form, taste, and texture[15]. Of note, special testing was conducted to confirm which children were impulsive. The table shows the foods that were used to provide variety, because if you're like me, and you read that impulsive children are more likely to overeat when presented with foods that varied in "color, form, taste, and texture", you want to know which foods those were! Other researchers confirmed that children and adolescents with ADHD tend to eat convenient and easily available foods that are high in fat and sugars[4] as they tend to choose the immediate choice[5]. Keep all of this in mind for the next chapter when we talk about the possible effect of artificial food colorings and sugar sweetened beverages on ADHD.

"Variety" Foods	"Monotonous" Foods
5 kinds of marshmallows: • white-pink marshmallows • pink marshmallows covered in coconut • white marshmallows covered in coconut • marshmallows covered in milk chocolate • yellow and green marshmallows in different forms	Only regular White/Pink Marshmallows

Prevention and/or management of overweight and obesity in children with ADHD should focus on management of food-related behaviors in addition to nutrient content of meals provided. This fact also promotes the idea that the healthy choice should be the easy and default choice in many food establishments, especially in hospital cafeterias and other healthcare settings.

An example of a "default choice" for healthy eating is when a hospital cafeteria uses a whole grain bun for a grill item unless the customer specifically asks for a white bun, and all pre-made deli sandwiches presented for sale are on whole grain, high fiber breads.

Once these children with ADHD start to take stimulant medications like methylphenidate, they are then actually more at risk of being <u>underweight</u> than overweight or obese. Stimulant medications are well-known for causing decreased appetite and weight loss[16]. This may be due to nausea and/or the fact that the medications stimulate neurotransmitter activity in the brain leading to a slow-burn type of "flight or fight" response. This chemical response from the neurotransmitters can lead to decreased appetite. Therefore, children with ADHD who have started on these medications have 1.6 times higher odds for being underweight compared to children without ADHD[14]. Tolerance to the medication side effects builds up over time in most people, which means that the appetite will eventually return. For the children who have reduced appetite from the medication, behavioral management related to food remains a key focus of treatment, in addition to the nutrient content of meals provided and the timing of meals and snacks in relationship to medication administration. Registered dietitians can focus education for parents on increasing the nutrient content of foods eaten while avoiding "empty calories" that contribute to satiety (a feeling of being full) but not nutrients needed for growth. As you guessed, I will provide strategies and tips for all of this in the next section.

Appetite and Medication Therapy

As discussed earlier, symptoms associated with ADHD can be caused by impaired neurotransmitter activity in the brain and medical treatment for ADHD usually involves treatment with methylphenidate or amphetamine-containing medications to repair this neurotransmitter activity. These medications are well-known appetite suppressants. Some children lose interest in eating altogether or won't eat at certain times of the day, and oral intake decreases significantly. Sometimes children adjust to the new medications and regain their appetite but others don't. This can lead to undesirable weight loss, and if this poor intake continues for several months it may affect growth in height and lead to micronutrient deficiencies with resulting medical issues. For example, if a child is not eating well and is losing weight, the overall intake of crucial nutrients for growth like iron and calcium is likely to be insufficient.

Some parents and children may choose to continue the medication regimen that causes the appetite suppression if the benefit of improved behavior outweighs the risk of decreased appetite. Therefore, dietitians should help these children and families with nutrition strategies to overcome the suppressed appetite before weight and/or growth are affected. A growth chart should be used to track weight and height over time, and discussed with the family and child to help guide decisions and the nutrition care plan.

Decreased oral intake should be discussed with the physician, as medication dosage and timing can be addressed to reduce the effects of appetite suppression. For example, methylphenidate is available in a long-acting formulation meant to be given one time per day, and in a short-acting formulation that is normally given two times per day. If appetite suppression continues for an extended period of time after starting the medication, instead of switching to a new medication, it may help to trial the same medication but in a different dosage or release rate. If this is not effective, and growth is negatively impacted, it may be necessary to change to a new medication altogether or even stop medication therapy.

A food frequency questionnaire, 24 hour diet recall, or other nutrition assessment tool should be used to evaluate the quality of the diet of the child as a first step, looking for particular areas of concern. For example, calcium intake may be insufficient if the child has decided not to consume any dairy products or iron intake may be insufficient if they have decided not to eat any meat. Recommendations for alternate food sources and/or supplementation can be made if needed. For other children, total intake of calories and protein and fluids may be significantly reduced, making it necessary to develop a more thorough approach to counteracting the effects of the appetite stimulation.

The registered dietitian should consult with the child's physician to determine if medication timing can be altered. If possible, breakfast should be provided before the first pill of the day, and should contain as many food groups as possible, with the child and family working with the dietitian to plan balanced meals. If the child is on a regimen that includes two pills per day, the second pill should be given after lunch. Similarly, the RD can provide balanced meal suggestions for lunch to maximize nutrient intake.

Many families are more willing to tolerate behaviors associated with ADHD when the child is at home, and are most concerned with using medication to help the child succeed at school or in activities outside the home such as organized sports or social settings. Therefore, the RD and family should consult with the physician on whether a "medication holiday" can be provided on weekends, holidays, and any other days in which the child will not be facing a challenging situation outside the home. This can allow for increased food and fluid intake on those days to compensate as much as possible for the days in which the child takes the medication and therefore does not eat as much.

In addition to possible alterations to medication timing and frequency, nutrition strategies are important. Foods and beverages chosen should be nutrient-rich, avoiding "empty calorie" foods such as soda, candy, or gelatin. Liquids should be offered between meals, rather than with meals or directly before the meal, in order to save appetite for solid foods. Behavioral strategies discussed in chapter _ of this book can also help improve intake in the child with decreased appetite.

Here is a sample meal and medication plan for a child

who takes a short acting medication two times per day and attends elementary school. Note: All medication plans must be approved by the child's physician.

7 am	Breakfast: Oatmeal made with milk and topped with raisins; hard-boiled egg.
7:30 am	1st medication dose
11:00 am	School lunch: Sandwich with whole grain bread (fortified with flax and Omega 3 fatty acids if possible) and extra peanut butter; banana or grapes, string cheese, milk
11:30 am	2nd medication dose (from school nurse)
2 pm	After school snack: Banana with peanut butter or Cheese and crackers
6:30 pm	Dinner: Chicken breast, steamed vegetable, baked potato with Omega 3 fatty acid-fortified margarine, milk

All fluids except for milk should be drank between meals rather than with meals to avoid filling the stomach with fluids instead of food. Just like with any other child, sugary beverages should be discouraged.

Austin had a decreased appetite during the first few weeks of taking methylphenidate. He said his friends were eating chocolate chip cookies, and he knew he would like them but he just didn't have any desire to eat them. He eventually adjusted to the medications and began to eat normally again. I have worked with a lot of other children who did not have improvement in appetite after being on the medications for any length of time. One child absolutely refused to eat anything at all on any days that she took any stimulant medication, but she also had very severe and disruptive ADHD behaviors when she was not taking medication. The parents, pediatrician, and her teachers worked together to determine which days she really needed the medication and which days she could skip the medication (including every weekend, holiday, and summer day) and provided as many nutrient rich foods as possible on those days.

KEY NUTRIENTS FOR GROWTH AND SPECIAL CONSIDERATIONS	
Calcium and Vitamin D	Healthy bones and teeth
Iron	Prevent anemia, promote growth
Water-soluble vitamins (Vitamin C and B vitamins)	Prevent infection and support metabolism; not stored in the body and therefore we need to consume daily.
Fat-soluble vitamins (Vitamins A, D, E, K)	Vitamin A – healthy skin, hair, and vision; Vitamin D – several functions, "sunshine vitamin"; Vitamin E – antioxidant; Vitamin K – necessary for blood clotting when injured. All of these vitamins require fat for absorption and are stored in the body so higher risk for toxicity when taken in high amounts.
Trace elements (Zinc, Copper, etc.)	Small amounts of these nutrients are required for growth and are stored in the body.
Macronutrients	Carbohydrate, Protein, and Fat All provide energy in the form of calories and are required for growth.

We have already talked a lot about "key nutrients for growth" and a "nutrient-rich diet" so this table provides a very brief overview of key nutrients and some helpful information about childhood nutrition related to these nutrients. The information here is not a comprehensive source of all the functions or sources of these nutrients but is meant more as an overview.

Artificial food colorings and preservatives

As a registered dietitian working with children and families who have either been referred by their pediatrician or primary care physician or are self-referred (asking to speak with me because of something they've read or heard or because they want to develop a nutrition plan for their child), I am often asked about the Feingold diet.

The investigation of the effect of artificial food colorings (AFCs) and preservatives and other food additives on childhood behavior was first popularized in the 1970s by Dr. Feingold when he published the Kaiser-Permanente diet[17]. He claimed that at least 50% of the children he worked with had improved behavior when omitting these foods from their diet. (Keep in mind, there were far fewer foods using these additives in the 1970s than there are now!) Many researchers then tried to test this diet, but these studies had the same challenges as those conducted on other food components and individual nutrients -- the results of one study did not always agree with the results of another. Outcomes of studies done comparing the behavior of children with ADHD when AFCs and/or food preservatives are eliminated from the diet is conflicting[18,19]. This is likely due to small sample sizes of children being studied, a big difference in the amount of AFCs and preservatives fed to the children, and a difference in whether the children in the study were actually diagnosed with ADHD or not.

For the healthcare professionals reading this, I will provide some details of the actual studies so that we can delve deeper into this popular and sometimes confusing issue. The total amount of AFCs certified by the FDA increased 5-fold from 1950 to 2012! The Food and Drug Administration (FDA) now limits the AFCs allowed in the U.S. diet to 9 different colors. AFCs are found in many beverages and some ready-to-eat cereals, popsicles, ice cream and sherbets, gelatin, puddings, cakes, cookies, boxed dinners, beverage syrups, snacks, and candy. Foods and beverages that are high in AFCs are also often high in sugar. Refer to an article published in Clinical Pediatrics in 2015 that contains tables listing the amounts of AFCs and sugar in several popular foods and beverages (reference 20).

Many foods that contain AFCs also contain food preservatives. Sodium benzoate is a food preservative that has been studied in relationship to hyperactivity, and is used in processed foods and soda to disrupt the growth of microorganisms (such as bacteria) that would otherwise cause the food to spoil. The FDA considers it a Generally Recognized as Safe (GRAS) substance because safety studies showed that at least 90 times the amount that is normally present in our diet would need to be consumed in order to cause any adverse health effects. Critics of the FDA's stance on sodium benzoate state that conclusion was made in 1973, and our food supply has changed drastically since then.

The Federal Food, Drug, and Cosmetic Act (FDC Act) states that any substance that is intentionally added to food is a food additive, but is not subject to premarket review and approval by FDA if the substance is generally recognized, among qualified experts, as having been adequately shown to be safe under the conditions of its intended use. These products are known as "GRAS" products, or "generally recognized as safe".

A 2007 study reported that a mixture of four AFCs plus the preservative sodium benzoate aggravated hyperactivity in two groups of children, 3 year olds and 8-9 year-olds without ADHD[19]. A second mix of AFCs didn't have as great an effect on the 8- to 9-year-olds, even though it also contained sodium benzoate and two of the same colorings, albeit in lower amounts. The assumption is made by many that the effect would be greater on children with ADHD, but this hasn't been confirmed with any studies that I could find. A different set of researchers in Hong Kong tested 130 children with an average age of 8 ½ years to see if AFCs and/or sodium benzoate would affect behavior[25]. They stated it was a "general population" which means they did not record whether the child had previously been tested for or diagnosed with ADHD. Two behavior scores were used to determine an effect, but neither mixture of AFCs and sodium benzoate had a significant adverse effect on the children.

An early behavioral study tested children with only about 27 mg of AFCs and reported that few children were sensitive to the AFCs[19]. Critics of that study stated that much larger doses of AFCs should have been used for the food challenges. Later studies used larger amounts and reported a higher percentage of children with adverse behavioral reactions to AFCs. For example, a study of 20 children reported that 17 of them reacted poorly on a learning task after consuming 100 to 150 mg of a mixture containing different AFCs[21]. Yet another study reported adverse reactions to a 125-mg mix of AFCs in 8 of 19 children (42%) based on standard parents' rating scales[22]. Two British studies measured the amount of behavioral changes in a large population of children consuming AFCs, using only 20 to 30 mg of AFCs (plus the preservative sodium benzoate) for the challenges[19,23]. They reported that the AFCs (and/or the sodium benzoate) did have an effect on the children's behavior.

One difficulty of studying the effects of AFCs and food preservatives on behavior and then translating that research into practical advice for the public, is that foods and beverages vary so widely in the combinations and concentrations of those substances. The Hawthorne effect discussed earlier will always affect these studies – the results are measured by someone's perception of behavior, and they almost always know an intervention has taken place. However, many advocacy groups repeatedly lobby the FDA to ban AFCs and sodium benzoate in the United States due to assumed adverse effects on children's behavior or their perceptions of their own child's behavior after eating or drinking foods with these substances.

BOTTOM LINE ON AFCs AND FOOD PRESERVATIVES: A small percentage of children will have improved behavior when AFCs and food preservatives are removed from the diet. This is a challenging diet to follow, and can be very restrictive. When consulted to determine whether to implement a diet eliminating these very prevalent food components to improve ADHD behavior, dietitians should have conversations with parents about the pros and cons of attempting this while managing other lifestyle and behavioral management components of ADHD. If the family does want to try to eliminate these substances, then an Elimination Diet trial is appropriate to determine if AFCs and/or food preservatives do influence that child's behavior.

Elimination Diet

We discussed in the last section the conflicting research surrounding AFCs and food preservatives on child and adolescent behavior. Even though there is not a lot of well-designed research that supports the use of elimination diets to treat ADHD, anecdotal online evidence reports improved behavior with children who followed an elimination diet to reduce or eliminate AFCs, food preservatives, and the foods Dr. Feingold recommended to avoid (which he termed antigenic foods).

For children who are suspected of being sensitive, or for patients or families who would like to try this diet based on Dr. Feingold's work, a trial period for eliminating antigenic foods, AFCs, and foods with additives may be warranted. Nutrition and medical professionals need to gain experience with these dietary preferences to properly oversee nutritional status and provide appropriate guidance to ensure the child meets nutrient needs for healthy growth and development despite the restricted diet.

An elimination diet is often used to determine which food is causing a bad reaction, such as a child who gets hives or other signs of allergic reactions after eating foods, but is having trouble distinguishing which food(s) is causing the problem. Skin prick tests for allergic reactions to foods are unreliable, and these reactions are better investigated with an elimination diet. An elimination diet can also help determine if avoiding certain foods will improve ADHD-related behavior.

Usually only 5-10 foods are allowed during the initiation phase, which should last 2-3 weeks. The foods allowed are the ones least likely to cause the reaction, and are never combination foods such as pizza or casseroles. If the initiation phase leads to a reduction of symptoms, then one new food is added back to the diet at a time, with a new food introduced every 3 – 5 days. When the symptoms return, then the most recently introduced food is identified as a culprit and eliminated again. This pattern repeats until all offending foods are identified. If the initiation phase of 2-3 weeks does not improve symptoms, then it is unlikely that diet is a contributing factor (assuming that adequate compliance to the diet is achieved) and the child can return to their usual diet. Obviously, this takes patience and diligence for both the parents, child, teachers, and anyone else who is involved in the eating environment for that child. Teachers and other caregivers should be notified about the diet to help improve compliance, or the diet should be done during summer or other school breaks when the food environment can be more easily controlled.

Listed in the table below are the specific foods to be avoided when following Dr. Feingold's Kaiser Permanente diet. When deciding which 5 – 10 foods will be allowed during the initiation phase of the elimination diet, the foods in the "Foods Allowed" column should be used, and food labels can help ensure avoidance of those versions with AFCs or food preservatives. Other family members may want to follow a similar diet at home to avoid making the child with ADHD feel isolated or singled out during meal times. Many of these foods, such as hot dogs and sugary beverages, are discouraged in overall healthy diets anyway. Special care will need to be given for food settings outside the home such as school, parties, and other social events. For example, pears and bananas are easy to pack and have ready for the child to eat when his or her peers are eating apples and grapes. However, some of the foods, such as apples and grapes, are foods that are often well liked by children, are included in many social occasions such as halftime at sporting events, and can be healthy snacks.

DR. FEINGOLD'S DIET	
Foods to Avoid	**Foods Allowed**
Apples	Grapefruit
Grapes	Pears
Luncheon meats	Pineapple
Hot dogs	Bananas
Cold drinks with artificial	Beef and lamb
flavors/colors	Plain bread
Red and orange synthetic	Selected cereals (without
dyes	dyes)
BHT and BHA food	Milk, eggs
preservatives	
Vitamins and medications	
with colorings	

In the studies reviewed in the previous section, it took 10 – 14 days to see a difference in behavior in the children for whom it was an effective intervention. Therefore, a minimum of a 2-to-3-week trial of this initiation phase of limiting the diet to 5-10 foods is necessary to determine if it will reduce ADHD symptoms. If behavior changes are not noticed within 3 weeks, then it is unlikely to make a difference – all healthy foods can be reintroduced and other interventions should be considered. If behavior is improved, the parents and child can reintroduce 1 of the restricted food items every 3-5 days. If the concerning behavior returns, then the reintroduced food is identified as an offender and should be avoided indefinitely.

A registered dietitian can help the family do a pantry and refrigerator analysis of all the foods currently in the home and make recommendations for healthy alternatives that fit within the elimination diet plan. He/she can help the family plan ahead for dining situations such as fast food or casual dining restaurants, social situations, and other food-related events. Vitamins and medications (and even toothpaste!) need to be evaluated for the presence of AFCs and preservatives as well, so families may need to consult a pharmacist for detailed information. Monthly visits with the registered dietitian are recommended until the diet is advanced to include more foods to evaluate diet intake records for nutritional adequacy, track anthropometric (growth) measurements, and make referrals to other healthcare professionals as needed.

Food Allergies & Hypersensitivities

Food allergies have been associated with behavioral and psychological symptoms, including those associated with ADHD[24,25]. Interestingly, psychosocial abnormalities have been reported to lead to food allergies as well[25]. Some reports show that allergic reactions during infancy can predict later neurodevelopmental abnormalities.[26] Overall, the research as to the prevalence of ADHD and allergic diseases can be conflicting[26-31], but the general consensus is that even if a relationship does exist, a cause and effect relationship cannot be established yet. In other words, it can't be determined if the factors that cause ADHD are the same factors that cause food allergies, or if food allergies or hypersensitivities cause ADHD symptoms.

It has been reported that up to 12% of children diagnosed with ADHD are using complementary and alternative medicine to treat the ADHD, such as using the elimination diets we just described and/or avoidance of hyperallergenic foods such as egg, seafood, milk, wheat, chocolate, and nuts[32]. Therefore, healthcare professionals should ask patients and families with whom they are working if they are using any dietary interventions to manage the ADHD and refer them to a registered dietitian if they are doing so. The dietitian should honor the family's preferences as much as possible, while working with them to create a nutritionally complete meal plan. The child can likely meet their nutrient needs if avoiding egg, seafood, milk, wheat, chocolate, nuts, or other allergens but it will be difficult.

<u>Sugar</u>

Sugar is popularly associated with behavior-related problems, like the hyperactivity and inattentiveness associated with ADHD. This may be partially related to the fact that many beverages with AFCs also have sugar. And traditionally, people have thought that eating or drinking sugar leads to hyperactivity. Sugar sweetened beverages (SSBs) account for about 80% of the total sugar consumed in this country, which is why most studies investigating the impact of sugar focus on SSBs.

Many studies investigating the impact of sugar intake on behavior also investigate the use of sugar substitutes[33]. Sugar substitutes include well-known brands like Splenda (sucralose), Equal (aspartame), or Sweet-n-Low (saccharin). Sugar substitutes are also known as artificial sweeteners or non-caloric sweeteners. They are many times sweeter than sugar, and therefore are needed in smaller amounts. They do not add calories to the diet, but many people have been concerned about these artificial sweeteners in the same way they are concerned about artificial food colorings or food preservatives.

A meta-analysis of 16 studies of sugar and sugar substitute intake in children with and without ADHD published in 1995 stated that there is no proof that sugar consumption causes hyperactivity[34]. The Academy of Nutrition and Dietetics issued a position statement in 2012[35] about the subject after a thorough review of the literature available at that time. Their conclusion was that sweeteners, whether real or artificial, do not affect the behavior of children with or without ADHD.

A study published in 2016 investigated the dose of sugar consumed from SSBs in children ages 4-15[36]. A strength of the study is that they only included children with doctor-diagnosed ADHD in the study group (i.e. did not include parent self-reported diagnosis) and had a decent size sample (101 kids with ADHD and 159 without ADHD in the control group). However, they did not report on whether the children were taking any medications to control ADHD nor did they report on the severity of symptoms. Their results showed that children who consumed 7 or more SSBs per week were almost 4 times as likely to have ADHD. There was no investigation on whether the intake of SSBs contributed to an increased severity of symptoms and did not establish a cause and effect relationship. In other words, there was no way to tell if the intake of SSB contributed to the behavior symptoms or if the fact that the children had ADHD made them more likely to drink SSBs. A full analysis of the diet showed that children with ADHD consumed 297 +/- 420 gm of sugar/week vs the 117 +/- 198 gm of sugar/week consumed by the other children, and that the children with ADHD also ate fewer fruits and vegetables than the children without ADHD.

| ADHD group: 297 +/- 420 gm of sugar/week |
| = <u>74 + /- 105</u> teaspoons sugar/week! |
| Control group: 117 +/- 198 gm of sugar/week |
| = 29 +/- 50 teaspoons sugar/week |

A larger study was published in 2015 that surveyed 1649 middle school students with an average age of 12.4 years[37]. Using a health behavior questionnaire and a hyperactivity/inattention questionnaire, the children themselves were asked to rate their own behaviors. They were then asked to list all of the SSBs that they had consumed in the last 24 hours. There was a strong correlation between high intake of SSBs and self-reported hyperactivity and inattention scores. Sixty-six percent of these middle school students said they had consumed at least one energy drink in that 24 hours, so the effect of the sugar could not be understood independently of the caffeine consumption. A limitation of this study is that one 24 hour period cannot be believed to be indicative of an overall diet pattern, and self-reporting of behaviors from children that young may not be accurate. Additionally, there was no investigation into whether any of these children had been diagnosed with ADHD or were taking behavior altering medications.

Many people ask 2 questions after hearing or reading all of this, and I will attempt to answer them here:

1. If science doesn't show a link between hyperactivity and sugar, why does my kid seem to get hyper when he has sugar?

➢ Consider the situations in which you allow a child to have sugar. It's usually for special occasions, like a birthday party or holiday. These are exciting times for kids! The stimulation involved in the event itself can increase the hyperactivity for a child with or without ADHD, and coincidentally increased sugar intake happens at the same time.

➢ For kids with ADHD who have trouble with sensory gating (aka filtering), controlling behavior can be even harder in these situations. He cannot filter out all that extra stimuli from the party, and that fact alone can cause him to become overwhelmed and act more aggressively or hyperactively.

➢ Many foods and beverages with sugar also have AFCs, so the behavior effects, if related to the foods/beverages, cannot be isolated to one component such as sugar.

➢ There's also the Hawthorne effect – a parent who gives their child sugar and then watches closely and expects to see altered behavior as a response is likely to see altered behavior. We often find what we're looking for.

2. If sugar doesn't cause ADHD or hyperactivity or inattention, why do kids with ADHD consume more sugar?

➤ Kids with ADHD are more impulsive, so they will often choose the immediate, easy, and gratifying choice. Sugar is everywhere in our food supply! There's usually a lot of sugar in foods and beverages that are brightly colored – these foods have been proven to attract kids with ADHD. So there are likely a lot of factors contributing to increased consumption of these foods and beverages by children with ADHD.

➤ I do want to share an interesting idea, though it is underdeveloped and not fully proven yet. A physician published this theory in a National Institutes of Health Open Access journal. It is very important to mention that this physician had a patent application on inhibition of fructokinase as a mechanism to treat sugar craving at the time of the publication, so that may have persuaded his theory. It is interesting nonetheless, and just food for thought for now in my opinion. He stated that ingestion of sugar increases dopamine for a short period of time, and therefore "children with ADHD may ingest more sugar than other children in an attempt to correct the dopamine-deficient state". In other words, children with ADHD may unknowingly reach for the SSBs or sugary food to correct the dopamine deficiency that is contributing to the ADHD. This theory needs more investigation to be proven, and since chronic sugar intake will lead to obesity, metabolic problems, and dental decay, allowing regular sugar intake is not a strategy that anyone would recommend to treat ADHD!

Austin was 10 in the summer after receiving his diagnosis. We had been talking about the research I was reading about nutrition and ADHD, and he knew that there is no proof that sugar causes hyperactivity. We lived in a small town in Virginia at the time, and went to the 4th of July parade with the neighbors. Austin's friends were eating the candy being thrown by the people on the parade floats, then running around, darting in between crowds of people and cars. He told his friends to stop acting crazy, and they told him "we can't help it, we've eaten too much candy!" Austin stood up tall, and in his 10-year-old voice said "You can't use that as an excuse. Sugar doesn't cause hyperactivity, you're just being wild. I know this because my mom is a dietitian!" I loved it!

BOTTOM LINE ON SUGAR: While there is no scientific proof that sweeteners increase hyperactivity, it is well known that excess sugar intake is not good for children or adults for a wide variety of other nutritional and dental reasons. Therefore, as health practitioners, we should always encourage decreased intake of simple carbohydrates and sugars, such as donuts, cakes, candies, white bread, etc. Instead, we should help parents, children, and others replace these simple carbs with whole grains and complex carbohydrates.

Simple Carbohydrates to avoid	Recommended replacements with complex carbohydrates
White bread	Whole grain bread (check food labels to ensure at least 3 gm fiber per slice)
White rice	Long grain brown rice, quinoa, farro
Any starch that boils in 3 minutes or less	Choose the longer cooking varieties as these have not used alkaline processing that breaks down the whole grains and fiber
White flour tortillas or buns	Whole grain tortillas or buns
White potatoes	Squash
Sugar sweetened cereals	Choose cereals with at least 3 gm fiber per ½ cup serving

Chapter 5 References

1. Ptacek R, Kuzelova H, Stefano G, et al. Disruptive patterns of eating behaviors and associated lifestyles in males with ADHD. *Med Sci Monit.* 2014;20:608-613.

2. Altafas JR. Prevalence of attention deficit/hyperactivity disorder among adults in obesity treatment. *BMC Psychiatry.* 2002;2:9-17. doi: 10.1186/1471-244X-2-9

3. Curtin C, Bandini LG, Perrin EC, Tybor DJ, Must A. Prevalence of overweight in children and adolescents with attention deficit hyperactivity disorder and autism spectrum disorders: a chart review. *BMC Pediatr.* 2005;5:48-55.

4. Donahoo W, Wyatt HR, Kriehn J, et al. Dietary fat increases energy intake across the range of typical consumption in the United States. *Obesity.* 2008;16;64–69.

5. Banaschewski T, Hollis C, Oosterlaan J, Roeyers H, Rubia K, Willcutt E. Towards an understanding of unique and shared pathways in the psychopathophysiology of ADHD. *Dev. Sci.* 2005;8; 132–140.

6. Poulton A. Growth on stimulant medication; clarifying the confusion: a review. *Arch Dis Child.* 2005;90:801-806.

7. Ptacek R, Kuzelova H, Paclt I, Zukov I, Fisher S. ADHD and growth: Anthropometric changes in medicated and non-medicated ADHD boys. *Med Sci Monit.* 2009;15:CR595-599.

8. Agranat-Meged AN, Deitcher C, Goldzweig G, Leibenson L, Stein M, Galili-Weisstub E. Childhood obesity and attention deficit/hyperactivity disorder: a newly described comorbidity in obese hospitalized children. *Int J Eat Disord.* 2005;37(4):357–359.

9. Holtkamp K, Konrad K, Mü¨ller B, et al. Overweight and obesity in children with attention deficit/hyperactivity disorder. *Int J Obes Relat Metab Disord.* 2004;28(5):685–689.

10. Lam LT, Yang L. Overweight/obesity and attention deficit and hyperactivity disorder tendency among adolescents in china. *Int J Obes.* 2007;31(4):584–590.

11. Bandini LG, Curtin C, Hamad C, Tybor DJ, Must A. Prevalence of overweight in children with developmental disorders in the continuous National Health and Nutrition Examination Survey 1999–2002. *J Pediatr.* 2005;146(6):738–743.

12. Troiano RP, Flegal KM. Overweight children and adolescents: description, epidemiology, and demographics. *Pediatrics.* 1998;101:497–504.

13. Hubel R, Jass J, Marcus A, Laessle RG. Overweight and basal metabolic rate in boys with attention deficit/hyperactivity disorder. *Eat Weight Disord.* 2006;11(3):139–146.

14. Waring ME, Lapane KL. Overweight in children and adolescents in relation to attention deficit/

hyperactivity disorder: Results from a national sample. *Pediatrics*. 2008;122:e1-e6. doi:10.1542/peds.2007-1955.

15. Guerrieri R, Nederkoorn C, Jansen A. The interaction between impulsivity and a varied food environment: its influence on food intake and overweight. *International Journal of Obesity*. 2008;32:708–714.

16. Methylphenidate. Medline Plus Web site. Available at http://www.nlm.nih.gov/medlineplus/druginfo/meds/a682188. html. Updated March 5, 2014. Accessed July 2, 2014.

17. Medical history scholar revisits KP allergist Feingold's hyperactivity diet. Kaiser Permanente Website. http://kaiserpermanentehistory.org/tag/feingold-diet/. Updated September 11, 2011. Accessed July 2, 2014.

18. Lok KYW, Chan RSM, Lee VWY, et al. Food additives and behavior in 8- to 9-year old children in Hong Kong: A randomized, double-blind, placebo controlled trial. *J Dev Behav Pediatr*. 2013;34:642-650.

19. McCann D, Barrett A, Cooper A, et al. Food additives and hyperactive behaviour in 3-year old and 8/9 year-old children in the community: a randomized, double-blinded, placebo-controlled trial. *Lancet*. 2007;370:1560–1567.

20. Stevens LJ, Burgess JR, Stochelski MA, Kuczek T. Amounts of artificial food dyes and added sugars in foods and sweets commonly consumed by children. *Clinical Pediatrics* 2015;54:309–321.

21. Swanson JM, Kinsbourne M. Food dyes impair performance of hyperactive children on a laboratory learning test. *Science*. 1980;207:1485-1487.

22. Pollock I, Warner JO. Effect of artificial food colours on childhood behaviour. *Arch Dis Child*. 1990;65:74-77.

23. Bateman B, Warner JO, Hutchinson E, et al. The effects of a double blind, placebo controlled, artificial food colourings and

benzoate preservative challenge on hyperactivity in a general population sample of preschool children. *Arch Dis Child.* 2004;89:506-511.

24. deTheije CGM, Bavelaar BM, da Silva SL, Korte SM, Olivier B, Garssen J, Kraneveld AD. Food allergy and food-based therapies in neurodevelopmental disorders. *Pediatr Allergy Immunol.* 2014;25:218-226.

25. Chida Y, Hamer M, Steptoe A. A bidirectional relationship between psychosocial factors and atopic disorders: a systematic review and meta-analysis. *Psychosom Med.* 2008;70:102–116.

26. Suwan P, Akaramethathip D, Noipayak P. Association between allergic sensitization and attention deficit hyperactivity disorder (ADHD). *Asian Pac J Allergy Immunol.* 2011;29:57–65.

27. Biederman J, Milberger S, Faraone SV, Lapey KA, Reed ED, Seidman LJ. No confirmation of Geschwind's hypothesis of associations between reading disability, immune disorders, and motor preference in ADHD. *J Abnorm Child Psychol* 1995;23:545–552.

28. Hammerness P, Monuteaux MC, Faraone SV, Gallo L, Murphy H, Biederman J. Reexamining the familial association between asthma and ADHD in girls. *J Atten Disord* 2005;8:136–143.

29. McGee R, Stanton WR, Sears MR. Allergic disorders and attention deficit disorder in children. *J Abnorm Child Psychol.* 1993;21:79–88.

30. Gaitens T, Kaplan BJ, Freigang B. Absence of an association between IgE-mediated atopic responsiveness and ADHD symptomatology. *J Child Psychol Psychiatry.* 1998;39:427–431.

31. Schmitt J, Buske-Kirschbaum A, Roessner V. Is atopic disease a risk factor for attention deficit/hyperactivity disorder? A systematic review. *Allergy.* 2010;65:1506–1524.

32. Sinha D, Efron D. Complementary and alternative medicine use in children with attention deficit hyperactivity disorder. *J Pediatr Child Health*. 2005;41:23-26.

33. Kruesi MJ, Rapoport JL, Cummings EM, et al. Effects of sugar and aspartame on aggression and activity in children. Am J Psychiatry. 1987;144(11):1487–1490.

34. Wolraich ML, Wilson DB, White JW. The effect of sugar on behavior or cognition in children. *JAMA*. 1995;274(20):1617-1621.

35. Position Paper. Position of the Academy of Nutrition and Dietetics: Use of nutritive and nonnutritive sweeteners. *J Acad Nutr Diet*. 2012;112:739-758.

36. Yu CJ, Du JC, Chiou HC, et al. Sugar-sweetened beverage consumption is adversely associated with childhood ADHD. *Int J Environ Research Public Health*. 2016;13:678-696.

37. Schwartz DL, Gilstad-Hayden K, Carroll-Scott A, et al. Energy drinks and youth self-reported hyperactivity/inattention symptoms. *Acad Pediatr*. 2015;15:297-304.

6 NUTRIENT SUPPLEMENTATION

Certain nutrients deserve special consideration when discussing nutrition and ADHD.

Omega-3 Polyunsaturated Fatty Acids (PUFAs)

First, I will provide a quick and simplified background on the different types of fats. They can all be put into 3 different categories – saturated, monounsaturated, and polyunsaturated fatty acids. Saturated fatty acids are typically thought of as "bad fats", while unsaturated fatty acids are considered "good fats". Omega 3 fatty acids are considered the healthiest polyunsaturated fatty acid (PUFA). From now on, I'll simply refer to them as Omega 3s. The abbreviated names of these Omega 3s are EPA, DHA, ALA (that is how they are most commonly referred to in the food marketplace and in studies). Omega 3s play an important role in neuron cell membrane elasticity and myelination and may affect neural signal transduction (the way brain cells communicate with each other). EPA regulates serotonin release (remember that neurotransmitter that we discussed in the diagnosis section? It's the one that has the most effect on executive function and sensory gating). While EPA regulates the release of serotonin, another kind of Omega 3 fatty acid called DHA is known to regulate the receptors that accept serotonin. So these 2 different types of Omega 3s have different and complementary actions – they help each other regulate serotonin!

Fast facts: The difference between saturated and unsaturated fats is the ratio of Hydrogen to Carbon molecules in their chemical chains. Saturated fats are completing "saturated" with hydrogen. This is why saturated fats are solid at room temperature while mono- and poly-unsaturated fats are liquid. Sometimes food manufacturers want to make polyunsaturated fats solid at room temperature (such as when making margarine) so they will add hydrogen across the double bonds. This can create a reaction that causes *trans*-fats, which are well known to contribute to heart disease.

Decreased blood levels of Omega-3s have been seen in those with ADHD[1,2]. Interestingly, women who consumed an omega-3 rich diet during pregnancy were less likely to have a child with ADHD-related behavior[3]. A Cochrane Review in 2012 concluded that there was limited data that symptoms were improved with the combination of omega-3 and omega-6 supplementation[4]. (Omega 6 fatty acids are another type of polyunsaturated acid.) Similarly, a meta-analysis conducted by Sonuga-Barke, et al.[5] showed that although statistically significant differences were seen in ADHD symptoms when children were supplemented with PUFAs, it was unclear how the supplements improved the behaviors and there was likely very little overall benefit to supplementation. Overall, while some studies that had been conducted up to that point did show that supplementation may lead to improvements in some aspects of ADHD behaviors, such as attention problems, other studies did not show this positive benefit, which led the Cochrane Review team to state that they could not make the recommendation for routine supplementation of Omega 3s to improve behavior[4].

The Cochrane Collaboration is a critically important source in evidence-based medicine – they provide scientific analysis of evidence to determine if a belief is based in science. Their goal is to help physicians and researchers make appropriate decisions about therapy, medications, or other healthcare interventions. Cochrane Reviews are systematic reviews of primary research in human health care and health policy, and are internationally recognized as the highest standard in evidence based healthcare.

Because of the increasing interest in the subject of Omega 3s for several different health outcomes, meta-analyses were then conducted in 2011 and 2013[1,6]. These came to similar conclusions as the Cochrane review: that there was likely very little clinical benefit to supplementation. Then in 2014, Barragan and colleagues[7] studied 90 children with ADHD in 3 groups: 1 treated with methylphenidate (more commonly known as Ritalin) alone, 1 treated with both Omega 3s and methylphenidate, and 1 group treated with only Omega 3s. The findings showed that the treatment was safe (which is the biggest question I ask as a mom!), and Omega 3s can effectively enhance treatment with methylphenidate by increasing the treatment effect, but that the treatment effect of Omega 3s alone was not comparable to that of medication. In other words, if a child's symptoms are being controlled with stimulant medications like methylphenidate, taking Omega 3 pills is not enough to replace those medications. But taking Omega 3s might help the medications be even more effective than they were before. The mechanism of action of this combination is unknown and is unlikely to be related to neurotransmitter receptor effects.

In 2015, a study was done with 40 boys with ADHD, ages 8 to 14, compared to a reference group of 39 boys without ADHD[8]. The children with ADHD either were not taking medications at all or were only taking methylphenidate, which is a stimulant medication. Changes in medication type or dosage were tracked throughout the 16 weeks of the trial as potential confounders. They were asked to eat 10 gms of fortified margarine per day, which is 2.2 tsp or just over 2/3 of a tablespoon. This margarine contained 650 mg of DHA and 650 mg of EPA. (Note: This was a specially fortified margarine for the study and might not reflect margarines that are bought in a grocery store.) This supplementation improved inattentiveness in boys with and without ADHD, which shows the importance of adequate intake of Omega 3 fatty acids during normal childhood growth and development even if the child does not have ADHD.

2011, 2012, 2013	Cochrane Review and 2 meta-analyses stated polyunsaturated fatty acids (mostly Omega 3s) improved symptoms but they were unclear how. "Likely very little clinical benefit to supplementation"
2014	Well-controlled study determined an Omega 3 supplement + methylphenidate increased benefit over methylphenidate alone
2015	Well controlled study determined the type and amount of Omega 3s is important -- Possibly need a supplement with both EPA and DHA 650 mg DHA and 650 mg EPA fortified margarine used for the study
2016 and beyond	??? I hope more research is done that helps determine the dosages and types of Omega 3s that have the most benefit while still being safe.

The table below lists the Omega 3 supplements that were studied in children with ADHD to determine efficacy and safety. This is not an exhaustive list of studies and only lists those with positive results. The goal is for the reader to determine minimum doses needed for a positive outcome (i.e. to control behavior) and the highest amount that has been studied for safety, in order to determine ideal supplementation doses if needed. Also, it is important to note that some of these supplements contained additional ingredients, such as Vitamin E or other types of Omega 3s besides DHA and EPA. Of course, any supplementation should be discussed with the child's physician to determine the appropriate dose and ensure supplements do not adversely affect any medications the child is taking.

Study	Doses; study length
Belanger et al, 2009[9]	500 – 1000 mg EPA and 100-400 mg DHA depending on the child's weight; 16 weeks
Bos et al, 2015[8]	Fortified margarine with 650 mg EPA and 650 mg DHA; 16 weeks
Stevens et al, 2003[10]	480 mg DHA and 80 mg EPA; 17 weeks
Richardson & Montgomery,2005[11]	558 mg EPA, 174 mg DHA; 26 weeks
Sinn & Bryan, 2007[12]; Sinn et al, 2008[13]	558 mg EPA, 174 mg DHA; 30 weeks
Johnson et al, 2009[14]	558 mg EPA, 174 mg DHA; 26 weeks

The next table below shows the foods that are high in Omega 3s – this is why the sample meal plan earlier in this chapter mentioned sandwich bread fortified with flax and Omega 3s! There are several good breads that are rich in fiber and Omega 3s by using flaxseed, but not all of them list the amount or type of Omega 3. This is the same situation with the fortified margarines. Therefore, if the food label does not clearly indicate the amount of DHA or EPA, the food should not be assumed to contain sufficient amounts of Omega 3s to have therapeutic effects on attention for children with ADHD.

FOOD SOURCES OF OMEGA 3S
Flaxseed
Walnuts
Chia Seed
Certain Cold Water Fatty Fish (Salmon, Mackerel, Trout)
Fortified eggs and margarines

OMEGA 3 CONTENT OF SUPPLEMENTS THAT CAN BE BOUGHT IN STORES

I'm not selling any of these, just providing information by reading labels on the supplements! I do not recommend one brand over another and there are more brands than what are listed here.

Brand	**Content per capsule/pill (compare these dosages to the studied amounts listed in the table above)**
GNC Triple Strength Fish Oil	EPA 734 mg DHA 267 mg "Other" 65 mg
Calamarine Omega 3	EPA 125 mg DHA 285 mg
NatureMade Fish Oil	EPA 360 mg DHA 300 mg "Other" 60 mg
Nordic Naturals Omega 3	EPA 165 mg DHA 110 mg "Other" 70 mg

This table shows the foods that are high in Omega 3s – this is why the sample meal plan earlier in this chapter mentioned sandwich bread fortified with flax and Omega 3s! There are several good breads that are rich in fiber and Omega 3s by using flaxseed, but not all of them list the amount or type of Omega 3. This is the same situation with the fortified margarines. Therefore, if the food label does not clearly indicate the amount of DHA or EPA, the food should not be assumed to contain sufficient amounts of Omega 3s to have therapeutic effects on attention for children with ADHD.

Of course people frequently ask me if I give Austin Omega 3s. He takes a low dose Omega 3 supplement even though I have never had him tested to see if he has low blood levels of Omega 3s. He rarely eats food sources of Omega 3s other than the fortified margarine that we all use at home and the bread he uses for sandwiches on school days. While the bread and margarine are fortified with Omega 3s, they are not EPA or DHA. He does not like nuts, and honestly, fatty fish like salmon is expensive and I don't do a good job cooking it at home. All of the studies show that the dosage of Omega 3s that he takes is safe over a long term basis. So, even if it doesn't make a difference for his ADHD behaviors, it isn't hurting him and it may help in other areas of health. Every time we run out of the bottle, we talk as a family with his physician to decide if we're going to continue it, and I check for any new research specifically related to safety levels of Omega 3 supplements.

BOTTOM LINE ON OMEGA 3s: Meta-analyses are finding some possible benefit to supplementing with Omega 3s, especially for improving attention, but better randomized controlled trial studies are necessary to determine if true effectiveness exists. The most promising results are shown when both EPA and DHA are supplemented, and supplementation up to 1 gm (1,000 mg) each of DHA and EPA appear to be safe for children. Dietitians should consider recommending supplementation with Omega-3s only when a deficiency is confirmed by a blood test or strongly suspected in the cases of limited dietary intake of PUFAs (see table for food sources) and only with the approval of the child's physician.

Practice Tips for Omega 3s Supplements:

➤ Does not replace medication therapy but may reduce dosage requirements or enhance the effectiveness of the medications.

➤ Most helpful for improving attention; may not help as much to reduce hyperactivity or impulsiveness.

➤ Need a supplement that has both EPA and DHA.

➤ Get advice from physician for dosages, especially with children. No need to use mega-doses! Most studied dosages are less than 1 gm of EPA and 1 gm of DHA.

➤ It seems safe to take Omega 3s for at least 26 weeks (6 months) according to the studies summarized in this chapter.

<u>Vitamin D</u>

Vitamin D is a fat soluble vitamin, which means when we eat foods with vitamin D we need to also eat something with fat so that it can be attached to fat to be absorbed in the intestine. It is also known as the sunshine vitamin, because when the ultraviolet B rays from the sun hit bare skin we make the active form of Vitamin D.

Fast fact: vitamin D metabolism is very complex – it involves different forms of the vitamin, and the kidneys, skin, and intestine all play different roles in vitamin D metabolism.

I'm sure many healthcare professionals reading this are now thinking "What is Vitamin D NOT linked to these days?" It is true that we are learning a lot more about the role of vitamin D in the body and its connection to various diseases when not available in adequate amounts or in the right metabolic forms. Many children with ADHD and other disorders associated with impulsive behavior have low blood levels of Vitamin D. Furthermore, supplementation in those individuals with low blood levels has been shown to improve inattention, hyperactivity, and impulsivity, which are the hallmarks of ADHD[15,16]! Most of the studies that supplement Vitamin D do so with 4,000 IU/day, but since this is a fat soluble vitamin that can be easily stored in the body, it is important to only supplement when a deficiency has been confirmed and only under the care and recommendation of a physician. I'd like to emphasize as well that 4,000 IU/day is not necessarily a mega-dose of a vitamin and it is not by itself meant to cure or treat ADHD.

Many people have asked me if Austin takes Vitamin D supplements. He is not taking them right now, mostly because I am worried about the cumulative effects of supplementing with a fat soluble vitamin that might build up in his blood and body. He also spends a lot of time in the sun without sunscreen on (unfortunately!) and we live in a part of the country that is sunny almost year round. He also drinks vitamin D fortified milk daily. I haven't had his serum Vitamin D levels tested, but I may consider it in the future and supplement if a deficiency is confirmed.

FOOD SOURCES OF VITAMIN D
Fatty fish, like tuna, mackerel, and salmon (these are also sources of Omega 3s!)
Foods fortified with vitamin D, like some dairy products, orange juice, soy milk, and cereals
Beef liver (Austin doesn't eat this!)
Cheese (One of Austin's favorite foods!)
Egg yolks

BOTTOM LINE ON VITAMIN D: If the child is confirmed to have low blood levels of vitamin D, talk with the physician about supplementation.

Practice Tips for Vitamin D Supplements:
- ➤ Check for deficiency first using a blood test.
- ➤ Possible recommended supplement dose is 4,000 IU/day (check with your physician!).
- ➤ Do not continue vitamin D supplements indefinitely; repeat blood test based on the schedule decided by the child's physician to determine if deficiency continues.

Other Micronutrients

Limited research has been done on blood levels of zinc, iron, and magnesium in children diagnosed with ADHD versus a control population without ADHD. Most studies show that these blood levels are lower in children with ADHD. Appropriate supplementation for children deficient in these nutrients produced small improvements in behavior, but only for those children with a deficiency confirmed with a blood test. These blood tests can be expensive, and children never like to be poked with a needle! I always encourage a full evaluation of the child's diet to determine if deficiency is likely before recommending a blood test to confirm. Dietitians should consult with the child's physician to develop an overall care plan, and supplement only children who have a verified deficiency. This is especially important since high amounts of one nutrient can interfere with the absorption of other nutrients (for example, calcium blocks the absorption of iron).

Even if deficiency of zinc, iron, or magnesium is verified and supplementation is started, the improvements in behavior are not likely to be enough to replace other interventions like medication, behavioral therapy, and supplements like Omega 3s. Since nutrient deficiencies should always be corrected, consult a physician to start supplementation of the appropriate nutrient. Recheck blood levels periodically to monitor the success of the supplementation and whether the supplementation can stop. Children and/or families following an elimination or restricted diet as treatment for ADHD should definitely consider having serum levels of these and perhaps other nutrients tested and supplement if needed as their diets are more likely to be limited in essential nutrients.

For the healthcare professional who is interested in a good overview of the research conducted on micronutrients related to behavior-related disorders, I recommend Natalie Sinn's article in *Nutrition Reviews* from 2008 (reference 17).

Chapter 6 References
1. Frensham LJ, Bryan J, Parletta N. Influences of micronutrient and omega-3 fatty acid supplementation on cognition, learning, and behavior: methodological considerations and implications for children and adolescents in developed societies. *Nutrition Reviews*.2012;70:594-610.

2. Richardson AJ. Omega-3 fatty acids in ADHD and related neurodevelopmental disorders. *Int Rev Psychiatry*. 2006: 18: 155–72.

3. Sagiv SK, Thurston SW, Bellinger DC, Amarasiriwardena C, Korrick SA. Prenatal exposure to mercury and fish consumption during pregnancy and attention-deficit/hyperactivity disorder related behavior in children. *Arch Pediatr Adolesc Med*. 2012: 166: 1123–31.

4. Gillies D, Sinn JKH, Lad SS, Leach MJ, Ross MJ. Polyunsaturated fatty acids (PUFA) for attention-deficit

hyperactivity disorder (ADHD) in children and adolescents (Review). *The Cochrane Library.* 2012;7:1-74.

5. Sonuga-Barke EJS, Brandeis D, Cortese S, et al. Nonpharmacological interventions for ADHD: Systematic review and meta-analyses of randomized controlled trials of dietary and psychological treatments. *Am J Psychiatry* 2013; 170:275–289.

6. Sonuga-Barke EJS, Brandeis D, Cortese S, et al. Nonpharmacological interventions for ADHD: Systematic review and meta-analyses of randomized controlled trials of dietary and psychological treatments. *Am J Psychiatry* 2013; 170:275–289.

7. Barragán E, Breuer D, Döpfner M. Efficacy and Safety of Omega-3/6 Fatty Acids, Methylphenidate, and a Combined Treatment in Children With ADHD. *J Atten Disord.* 2016;21: 433 – 441.

8. Bos DJ, Oranje B, Veerhoek ES, Van Diepen RM, et al. Reduced symptoms of inattention after dietary omega-3 fatty acid supplementation in boys with and without Attention Deficit/Hyperactivity Disorder. *Neuropsychopharmacology.* 2015;40:2298–2306.

9. Bélanger SA, Vanasse M, Spahis S, et al. Omega-3 fatty acid treatment of children with attention-deficit hyperactivity disorder: A randomized, double-blind, placebo-controlled study. *Paediatr Child Health.* 2009;14:89-98.

10. Stevens L, Zhang W, Peck L, et al. EFA supplementation in children with inattention, hyperactivity, and other disruptive behaviors. *Lipids.* 2003;38:1007–1021.

11. Richardson AJ, Montgomery P. The Oxford-Durham study: a randomized, controlled trial of dietary supplementation with fatty acids in children with developmental coordination disorder. *Pediatrics.* 2005;115:1360-1366.

12. Sinn N, Bryan J. Effect of supplementation with polyunsaturated fatty acids and micronutrients on learning and behavior problems associated with child ADHD. *J Dev Behav Pediatr.* 2007;28:82-91.

13. Sinn N, Bryan J, Wilson C. Cognitive effects of polyunsaturated fatty acids in children with attention deficit hyperactivity disorder symptoms: A randomised controlled trial. *Prostaglandins, Leukotrienes and Essential Fatty Acids.* 2008;4-5:311-326.

14. Johnson M, Ostlund S, Fransson G, Kadesjö B, Gillberg C. Omega-3/omega-6 fatty acids for attention deficit hyperactivity disorder: a randomized placebo-controlled trial in children and adolescents. *J Atten Disord.* 2009;12:394-401.

15. Patrick RB, Ames BN. Vitamin D and the omega-3 fatty acids control serotonin synthesis and action, part 2: relevance for ADHD, bipolar disorder, schizophrenia, and impulsive behavior. *FASEB J.* 2015;29:2207-2222.

16. Kamal M, Bener A, Ehlayel MS. Is high prevalence of vitamin D deficiency a correlate for attention deficit hyperactivity disorder? *Attn Defic Hyperact Disord.* 2014;6(2):73-78. doi: 10.1007/s12402-014-0130-5.

17. Sinn N. Nutritional and dietary influences on attention deficit hyperactivity disorder. *Nutrition Reviews.* 2008;66:558-568.

7 NUTRITION RECOMMENDATIONS TO COMPLEMENT BEHAVIOR MANAGEMENT FOR CHILDREN WITH ADHD

Behavior Management Overview

Evidence-based family training typically begins with weekly group sessions of about 10 weeks duration with a trained therapist or certified instructor. The focus is educating the parents (and child if age appropriate) about ADHD, and providing guidance to manage the child's behavior problems and difficulties in family relationships if they exist. These behavioral therapy programs offer specific techniques for reinforcing positive behaviors and decreasing or eliminating inappropriate behaviors, to help the child control their activity and impulsivity and improve attention. These programs emphasize establishing positive interactions between parents and children by

✓ learning how to shape children's behaviors through combinations of praising and ignoring
✓ giving successful commands
✓ identifying which behaviors are handled most appropriately through punishment and determining how to carry punishments out in a responsible and effective way.

These programs all emphasize teaching self-control and

building positive family relationships.

The behavioral therapy principles shared in these programs can also be applied to improving the way the child interacts with their food environment. In a previous chapter we discussed the eating behaviors displayed by children with ADHD, including impulsive food choices and eating as a distraction. Since there is a strong genetic component to ADHD, many times one or more family members have these same challenges. That is why it is important to work with the family members all together to develop coping strategies. Behavioral therapy is much more effective if those who are influential in the child's life are following similar principles.

I can't emphasize enough the importance of establishing routines and expectations that children need to follow, especially those with ADHD. It helps them to remember important things like where to put their homework, the self-care steps needed to get ready for school, and when it is or is not time to eat. Helping children with ADHD manage behaviors surrounding food and nutrition is important. Since the recommended food-related behaviors are also overall healthy behaviors, these should be encouraged for the entire family and children without ADHD.

Here are tips to establish and carry out a successful behavior management plan to help your child as shared by Beth Orenstein on Everyday Health[1].

- **Define the rules.** Make them simple and define the consequences (what will happen when the rules are obeyed and when they are not). Repeat them often. The rules need to be the same for every child in the house, not just the one with ADHD.

- **Give immediate and frequent rewards and consequences.** Children with ADHD need more immediate and frequent feedback for both their good and bad behavior than other children due to their need for immediate gratification. As the ADHD symptoms become more controlled, and the feedback becomes more consistent, it can happen less frequently.

- **Be consistent.** Reacting in the same way every time your child behaves in a positive or negative way helps your child know what to expect and believe that the rules are meant to be obeyed.

- **Establish routines.** Routines are important for every child, as they help him/her to feel secure that they can count on things to happen in a certain way at a certain time, and remember everything that needs to be done. This is even more important for children with ADHD. Establish everyday routines for getting ready for school, doing homework, and going to bed. A routine doesn't mean that everything has to happen at exactly the same time every day, but things still need to be scheduled in the same order. For example, the morning routine may consist of eating breakfast, taking medications, brushing teeth and putting on deodorant, packing the backpack with items needed for the day, and grabbing lunch on the way out the door, in that order. *We actually found that once we had settled on a good routine with Austin, if we threw in a reminder to do one of the steps (such as get his lunch from the refrigerator), it caused him to be more likely to miss a step. It was almost like we were inserting something different into the process that messed up the routine. Before he had even been diagnosed with ADHD, we learned how important routines were for him at bedtime. He simply could not fall asleep unless he had said bedtime prayers with both parents, and the prayer always had to end with the same sentence "Thank you Jesus for dying on the cross and rising off, Amen". If one of us was out of town for work, we had to be sure we called at bedtime to say the prayer, and not get off the phone until that closing sentence was said.*

- **Create checklists.** One way of getting a child to follow a routine is to have them create a checklist (if they're old enough to read and write) and mark off the steps as they are completed – this gives them a sense of control and ability to monitor their own activities without feeling like they're being micromanaged by a parent.

- **Set clocks and timers.** Establish times for key activities — when the family will have dinner, start homework, catch the school bus, stop watching TV, or get ready for bed — and set an alarm to signal each one. That way you don't have to stand over your child and nag. Also, you're clear and consistent about your child's schedule, with more clear guidance than saying "We'll do this in a few minutes." Many parents of children with ADHD have told me that setting a timer for when activities will start has been very beneficial for them. The child does not need to frequently ask when something will happen, because they can check the timer that is counting down. It also helps keep the parent accountable to the child and themselves, so that "we'll do this in a few minutes" doesn't turn into hours later due to getting distracted by other tasks.

- **Focus on the positive.** Emphasize the things that your child does right. For example, if given a multi-part task, say "good job" when she has completed the first part and be patient to explain the next step again if needed. Focusing on the positive, rather than berating her for not finishing the entire task, is more effective for a child with ADHD. This helps build confidence in her abilities. But always be genuine and provide praise only when it is due.

- **Plan for problems.** Many parents of children with ADHD can predict when their child is likely to be disruptive and misbehave, such as in exciting situations or when they're likely to be bored. If you can anticipate problems, use it to your advantage. Develop a plan for what you will do if your child misbehaves, especially in public, and share your plan with your child ahead of time. Making the child aware of consequences may lessen the likelihood that the behavior will occur. If your child does misbehave, remember your plan and follow through. Consistency is key!

- **Create a reward system.** Many times you can manage the behavior of children with ADHD with tokens that the child can trade for a special reward. *We set up such a system with Austin for the first few months after the diagnosis. Using Connect 4 game pieces (because they were two different colors), we established tasks that were worth a black piece (2 points) and tasks that were worth a red piece (4 points). If he completed the task, he got the appropriate game piece that he placed in a clear vase (so that he could see his pieces piling up). We assigned point values to certain rewards. On the next page is an abbreviated version of the table that we used. We only continued this system for a couple of months, because we found that it was effective for getting him on track, but after a few months when it lost its novelty he felt like he was being singled out (as compared to his brother). He also didn't want other people to visit the house and ask about the Connect 4 pieces in the vase. But most importantly, we found that providing praise and encouraging words in response to his positive behaviors were more effective than this reward system because he cared about us and how his behavior impacted us.*

Tasks worth a black game piece (2 points)	Tasks worth a red game piece (4 points)	Rewards (with points required to earn them)
Turn in math homework	Complete entire week at school with no reports about excessive talking	Trip to the skateboard park (15 points)
Clean the dinner dishes without being asked	Cook dinner	University of Virginia football tickets (25 points)
Desk is clean on random spot checks	Entire room is clean on random spot checks	Mom would do one of his chores for him (10 points)
Did not forget his lunch for an entire week	Every piece of homework turned in on time for the week	Brother would play a video game of his choice with him (15 points) – (He usually saved his points for this each time!)

This next section will focus on translating these great tips into successful nutrition strategies for children with ADHD. Many children without ADHD would also benefit from these strategies!

NUTRITION-RLEATED BEHAVIOR MODIFICATION

Avoid using food as a distraction.

Children with ADHD are impulsive and sometimes are described as "being driven by a motor". They can have a hard time focusing, and bounce from one activity to another. Many times parents learn that offering food can be a way to get a child to sit still even for a few minutes, which can be a very welcome relief for the parent. I think this is why grocery stores offer cookies to kids while the parents shop, so that they'll spend more time in the store and buy more (I'm pleased to see more grocery stores now offering free fruit for children instead of cookies). However, this can encourage the child to develop an unhealthy relationship with food, as the child may learn to eat whenever he/she is bored or expect to be entertained with food. Additionally, the child is likely to learn that "acting out" will be rewarded with food, and may therefore do so more frequently.

Instead of offering food as a distraction, many behavioral therapists will recommend providing positive reinforcement when the behavior is controlled. If a child does sit quietly and still in the grocery cart or at the doctor's office, the parent could provide positive encouragement every couple of minutes. For example, after 3 minutes of sitting quietly, the mom can say "thank you for being so well behaved," and a few minutes later, if still sitting appropriately, she can say "it makes my day so much easier when you sit still and quiet in these types of places". Keeping the child aware of how much longer the wait will be and all the activities that will need to happen prior to getting to be loud and moving again, will help the child understand and hopefully meet expectations.

Food as Rewards

Behavioral training programs for ADHD often involve establishing a positive reward system when the child demonstrates good behavior (see the sidebar above). Food should not be used as a reward or a punishment for any child, especially those with ADHD, because this can lead to negative associations surrounding foods that can be detrimental long term. Rewards could be activities or experiences rather than food.

Social outings

Social events, such as a dinner party or a visit at a friend's house, can bring additional challenges to a child with ADHD. New environmental stimuli, especially if unfamiliar, can increase the frequency and severity of symptoms, which can be stressful for the entire family. Parents should be encouraged to have a discussion with their child before going to social events. In addition to setting expectations for behavior management, parents should tell the child ahead of time which food choices will be acceptable, the planned eating schedule for the event, and when permission should be requested for deviations from the plan. For example, will the dinner be served family-style with common serving bowls, or will it be a formal plated dinner? Will the child be allowed to choose from a variety of offerings, or will he/she be expected to eat whatever is served? Of course, it is not always possible to know ahead of time the details about the food, so families can outline expected behavior with a variety of possibilities. Most importantly, the communicated plan must be enforced by the parents once at the social event; otherwise, the child will learn to circumvent the guidelines, leading to increasing difficulty to manage symptoms. Siblings should be expected to follow the same rules, because these are healthy food and social behaviors that would be beneficial for all children, regardless of ADHD diagnosis. This also helps the child to avoid feeling singled out or treated differently due to his diagnosis.

<u>"No" means no.</u>

Most children repeatedly ask for the same thing if it is highly desired, even if the parent has already said "no". This is likely to be amplified in the child with ADHD due to the tendency towards impulsivity and difficulty with delayed gratification. If a parent eventually gives in and changes "no" to "yes" with repeated questioning, children will learn to continually repeat the same question or request because they know they will eventually get the answer they want. This can be exhausting for the parent, and can lead to poor choices. Therefore, it is important for a parent to only say "no" when he/she really means "no", and then to stick with it. This is an important management technique for all behaviors, including those related to food.

Here is a story from a family I worked with whose 9 year old daughter had ADHD: Kelly would watch cartoons and see advertisements for foods during the commercial breaks. She would repeatedly ask her mom to go to the store to buy the food, but her mom would always say no because it was usually sugar sweetened cereals or beverages. During grocery store trips, Kelly would repeatedly ask for those foods again. One evening, Kelly's older sister was at the store with them, and asked for the same cereal. Her mom was especially tired that night, and bought the cereal in a moment of weakness. Kelly then knew that she could ask her sister to make the requests, and mom would be more likely to give in. The repeated requests continued, because Kelly had learned that "no might not always mean no". Her mom and I worked on a plan to determine which foods really needed a "no", and which foods could be given a "sometimes" designation, and to provide Kelly and her sister an explanation that buying the food one time did not mean that she would buy it on a regular basis. Resetting and reminding behavior expectations every few months is a very important management strategy with children.

<u>Make the healthy choice the easy choice.</u>

Since children with ADHD have an even harder time delaying gratification than others and will often choose the most convenient foods, it helps to make the healthy choice be the easy choice. For example, ready to eat, finger food snacks that are available in the house and in the school lunchbox or backpack should contain fruits and vegetables that are age appropriate. Ziplock baggies prepared with carrots or grapes are good examples, rather than chips or candy. Yogurt or cheese cubes can provide calcium as part of a healthy snack. Nuts are a good source of protein and Omega 3s, and are easily transported to activities outside of the home. Some children are more sensitive to textures of foods, so a variety of foods may need to be trialed. Unhealthy processed foods like chips, candy, and sugar sweetened beverages should not be kept around the house regularly – the family can enjoy them during special occasions outside the home!

This is also a reason to encourage population health management strategies in the community. School events, public eating venues like hospital cafeterias, grocery stores, state office buildings, and other community eating settings should practice the same concept of making the healthy choice the easy choice. For example, stores and cafeterias can establish a healthy registers policy – only food meeting pre-established criteria for "healthy" can be placed within 5 feet of the cash register, since this is where most last minute and impulse buys take place.

Meal times

Many times a diagnosis of ADHD, and therefore treatment, is delayed due to lack of recognition of symptoms and/or lack of access to medical care. In these cases, the family may have already found meal time to be challenging and made adjustments to the meal schedule, location, and/or content.

Just as behavioral management training for children with ADHD emphasizes the importance of establishing routines for the child for schoolwork, homework, and other aspects of behavior, routines should be established surrounding mealtime. Distractions at mealtimes, such as television or other electronic media, should be minimized as these children have a reduced ability to filter out distractions to concentrate on the task at hand. Children should be encouraged to chew slowly and really taste their food. If possible, movement should not be completely restricted at mealtime. While the child should not be allowed to get up from the table and wander around, if a bench can be substituted for a chair at the dinner table, movement can be allowed within a reasonable limit. This allows the child to concentrate on eating rather than being overly mindful of his movements or getting in trouble for moving too much. Establishing a family meal schedule at roughly the same time and same location each day can help the child know when and where to expect to eat. Snacks should also be planned, with limitations placed on eating between these scheduled times. This can help the child avoid eating as a distraction or out of boredom, and overall nutrient content was found to be better in children with ADHD who ate 3 meals with 0-2 snacks/day rather than being allowed to "graze" all day by eating small portions but eating almost constantly throughout the day.

Most children have a hard time waiting for dinner to be cooked, and this is especially true for children with ADHD who are impulsive and crave immediate gratification. Engaging the child in planning and cooking the meal can keep him/her involved in the process, and the child who is helping to cook the meal knows when it will be time to eat with an appreciation of the multiple steps involved.

While it's true that impulsivity, inattentiveness, and hyperactivity are each hallmarks of ADHD, so are creativity, innovation, imagination, and usually intelligence! Children with ADHD are often the best little chefs if this imagination and creativity are fostered correctly - Austin has actually become our family chef! I think his creative and imaginative mind allows him to think up new ways to cook the same foods, and his propensity towards math, science, and engineering contribute to him understanding recipe calculations and the science of food. He's often willing to cook dinner, IF I allow him to do it all by himself and allow him to cook from scratch rather than starting with packaged items. He's always asking why certain ingredients are needed or what role the egg, baking powder, baking soda, or whatever ingredient plays in the final product. As a registered dietitian, I should know the answers to all of those food science questions, but sometimes he stumps even me! Thankfully, many cookbooks will explain food science or he can look things up on the internet.

Working with my son in the kitchen has taught me several things that are helpful for all children, and not just those with ADHD:

- Children are known to ask (sometimes repeatedly) "when will dinner be done?" For children with ADHD and other behavioral diseases characterized by impulsivity, it is especially difficult for them to wait for the meal (or really anything else). But when they are helping make the food, they don't need to ask – they will know. Preparing the ingredients, assembling the meal, and placing it in the oven while setting the timer for cook time will give them something active to do while waiting and give them control and knowledge over the time to completion.

- All children are more likely to eat new foods if they help prepare them. Developmentally and age appropriate tasks should be assigned to children to help with some aspect of meal preparation, even if it is simply setting the table, washing the vegetables, or slicing the bread with a butter knife.

- Creativity and imagination should be encouraged, even in the cooking process! Let children experiment with new or substituted ingredients, just so they can see what will happen. Some of these are tried and true things, like substituting applesauce for the fat source in muffins to reduce the overall calories. While it's a well-known cooking trick for those of us who have been cooking for years, it is still a fun novelty for children while sneaking some "stealth health" into the food. Other times, let them try things that will have unexpected results (like using baking soda instead of baking powder to see for themselves the difference between the two, or using different spices and seasonings). If the meal doesn't turn out right, you can always have a back-up soup or crock-pot meal that can stand in its place. But the memories created, knowledge gained, and creativity fostered are priceless in comparison.

Family mealtimes are an excellent time for family conversations. Many children with ADHD, due to the associated impulsivity, have a hard time avoiding interrupting other people who are speaking, and/or changing the conversation topic abruptly. Because of the difficulty with concentration, they will often say that they know they'll forget what they wanted to say if they don't say it right away – which is why they interrupt. Or, they are not concentrating on the conversation being held by the rest of the participants, which is why they change the subject abruptly. Both of these habits can lead others to avoid conversations with these children, which can leave the child feeling sad and isolated without fully being able to understand why.

Rules should be established for conversations, especially mealtime conversations. Children should be reminded to not talk with food in the mouth, and not interrupt or change the subject, to help the child learn how to participate in mealtime conversations outside the home. Most behavioral therapists will agree that children with ADHD thrive on positive reinforcement rather than negative consequences – so the child should receive positive encouragement words when he goes even 3 minutes without interrupting at meals. If this positive feedback becomes routine, you will find that you can go longer between providing the feedback because the interrupting will decrease.

Eating outside the home

Buffets create a challenge for any impulsive person, especially when that impulsivity is manifested in eating behaviors. Since impulsivity is a trademark of ADHD and also can be typical of children in general, children and adolescents with poorly controlled ADHD are at particular risk for overeating when faced with buffets. This is especially true when the buffets include a dessert bar and/or fatty & fried food selections, as high fat and high sugar foods tend to be highly palatable, colorful, and inviting. Dietitians can recommend avoidance of buffets as much as possible, but should also provide strategies for helping families manage this environment for the occasions that a buffet is chosen.

Children should be supervised when serving themselves on the buffet. Portion sizes should be small, as the child can go back for seconds if they decide. Exploration of new foods should be encouraged, and selection of foods can be made into a game – for example, the child could be challenged to see how many different colors of foods he/she can put on their plate or to make a smiley face with vegetables on his plate. Dessert bars should be saved for last, and serving sizes should be kept small. The impulsivity can lead to excess eating at a buffet, as the person with ADHD will likely eat rapidly in order to return to the buffet to see what else is there. Children should therefore be encouraged to chew slowly and really taste their food, providing the opportunity for the "stomach to catch up to the eyes". All children can be asked to wait for a return trip to the serving stations until everyone at the table is ready for seconds to slow the pace of the meal. Plates with unwanted food should be cleared promptly to avoid the mindless eating that is common in these situations.

While most dietitians would prefer that children avoid fast food restaurants altogether, the reality is that many families eat at these restaurants anyway. Recommendations can be made on how to make healthier choices at these restaurants by reviewing nutrition information that is posted either in the restaurant or online. Children (and adults!) can be asked to choose fewer food items at the restaurant with the encouragement of adding a piece of fruit as a snack when returning home. Sugar sweetened beverages should never accompany a meal for children (or really adults either!) so fast food meal combinations are not recommended. Request water instead.

Sporting events such as a baseball or basketball game should not include trips to the snack bar, so that children will not always associate these types of events with food. Of course, if meals are missed or the game is long enough to allow the child to truly become hungry, the healthiest choice possible should be made at the snack bar. This would include a bottled water instead of a soda or other sugar sweetened beverage.

<u>Grocery Stores</u>

Taking a child with ADHD to any kind of store can be challenging, but this is especially true at the grocery store. Foods are marketed and displayed in the store to grab attention to the sale items and/or foods from which the manufacturers make the most profit. Unfortunately, these are usually highly processed foods full of sugar, fat, and sodium. Since children with ADHD have a reduced capability of filtering out external stimuli, they are typically drawn straight to these foods with colorful packages and may make multiple requests to purchase them. This would be another time when it is important to follow the idea that "no means no" – if the answer is "no", then that must be repeated every time the child asks (which will be frequent, especially if these foods are placed near the cash registers).

There are strategies for navigating the grocery store with a child with ADHD. Have the child help make a grocery list ahead of time, so that he/she knows those are the only items that will be bought. The grocery list can be divided into categories mirroring the food guide pyramid for an additional education moment, such as putting all dairy products together and all protein foods (such as lean meats, eggs, and nuts) into one section of the list. Foods that are considered staples, such as flour, butter, and milk, can be listed as such with a discussion about what this means. Let the child peruse the produce section and encourage the child to choose a new fruit or vegetable he/she hasn't tried previously, or perhaps to choose one fruit or vegetable from each color in the rainbow. All kids like games, and these types of games can help the ADHD child focus on a task at hand. If age appropriate and/or an older sibling can accompany the child, give him/her specific items on the shopping list to find in the store so that he/she has a sense of purpose during the trip. Another idea that includes a nutrition education component is to have the child choose an item, such as spaghetti sauce, based on the lowest sodium content or some other factor. Again, these are strategies that give a specific purpose to the trip for the child and help to foster a sense of independence.

A food staple is a food that makes up a large part of a population's diet, is eaten regularly, supply a major proportion of a person's nutritional needs, and are often used to prepare other foods. They vary from place to place and culture to culture, depending on the food sources available. In my family, food staples are milk, eggs, certain spices and seasonings, Smart Balance margarine (seriously, I use it daily and almost can't eat grains without it), whole grain bread, and peanut butter. If we're running to the store late at night, it's because we're out of one of these staples that is preventing us from finishing the meal we wanted to cook or because we will need it for breakfast.

Eating at School

School eating environments can often be challenging for students with ADHD. There is usually limited time for school lunches, and this time is shortened even more if the student needs to first go through a cafeteria line to get the lunch. Children with ADHD often have trouble waiting their turn, standing in a line, and need extra space in general. They also have trouble "delaying gratification", which in this case would involve waiting for their lunch to be served. Many times, the children eat inside a cafeteria with long rows of benches and tables, students squeezed in tightly together (creating less space), and there are a lot of distractions and noise that can be overwhelming to a student with ADHD. Many children with ADHD also complain about the sound of children chewing near them, even if those children are chewing quietly.

If possible, children with ADHD or any other disability should never be singled out at school in any way, as the extra attention can only serve to distract them more and stigmatize them. Whenever possible, students with ADHD should have the option to be excused for lunch a few minutes before the other children to allow extra time to get set up for lunch or get a place in line near the front of the serving line. They should also be allowed to sit on the end of the benches or at outside tables where they can stand up and move around within a reasonable structure. If the student prefers to blend in and sit in the middle of other students and not eat, then the teachers and school staff should notify the parents and allow them to make up for the missing nutritional value with a more substantial breakfast and after school snack.

Chapter 7 Reference

1. 10 ADHD Behavior Management Strategies. Everyday Health website. Available at http://www.everydayhealth.com/hs/adhd-and-your-child/adhd-behavior-management-strategies/. Updated July 8, 2010. Accessed March 27, 2017.

8 EXERCISE AND ADHD

Every child benefits from regular physical activity, whether or not they have ADHD! Specific benefits for the child with ADHD include the effect of exercise on tryptophan and serotonin (tryptophan is a precursor for serotonin). Exercise increases tryptophan transport across the blood-brain barrier, and increases serotonin production. It can also increase dopamine and norepinephrine production and possibly other neurotransmitters.

> Any amount of any kind of exercise shows measurable effect on neurotransmitters.

Even short term exercise results in improved cognition (brain function) and those who exercise regularly show a reduction in diseases that would cause brain problems. Sustained exercise like long runs create increases in serotonin and norepinephrine levels, which can lead to feelings of happiness and energy and increased executive brain functions. Since ADHD is a brain disease that decreases executive function in the brain and is related to decreased serotonin and dopamine levels, it is obvious that exercise can improve symptoms associated with ADHD due to the effects listed here. It is important to note that the effects of exercise on ADHD symptoms were found to be independent of methylphenidate action or use. In other words, exercise can improve ADHD symptoms if the child is taking medications to control the ADHD or if they are not.

According to a study published in 2003 in the *Journal of Applied Physiology*[1], researchers found that dopamine levels were raised during prolonged exercise but the levels returned to normal quickly. This explains why allowing an extra physical activity period for children with ADHD to "get the wiggles out" is not effective – the movement effects to stimulate dopamine release would be lost by the time the child returned to class. However, since any movement stimulates dopamine release, which can improve attentiveness and executive function for every child, it makes sense to allow children the freedom of movement to the greatest degree possible in the classroom environment. Thankfully, this has become more recognized and teachers are beginning to get standing desks and exercise balls for children to use instead of chairs, and allowing children to self-select seating arrangements to complete school work within reasonable accommodations.

There are multiple other benefits from exercise of course, as all children can use exercise to help maintain a healthy weight, and this remains true for children with ADHD.

Chapter 8 Reference
1. Nybo L, Nielsen B, Blomstrand E, Moller K, Secher N. Neurohumoral responses during prolonged exercise in humans. *J Appl Physiol.* 2003;95:1125-1131.

CONCLUSION

The nutrition-related research to improve symptoms associated with ADHD is new, exciting, and evolving! Healthcare professionals, parents, and caregivers can encourage healthy eating behaviors that are important for all children with a special focus on certain nutrients like Omega 3s and vitamin D. Behavioral management techniques can be used to improve the food environment and interactions with food, and the entire family can implement these same healthy eating behaviors as the child with ADHD.

Review of Key Points for Nutrition Management

✓ Impulsivity, inattentiveness, and hyperactivity are the main symptoms of ADHD. Nutrition strategies are aimed to improve one or more of these symptoms. No nutrition strategies can cure ADHD.

✓ Sugar does not increase hyperactivity, but for many other reasons all children, including those with ADHD, should be provided with a balanced, healthy diet with limited sugar content.

✓ Some children will benefit from following an elimination diet with gradual reintroduction of foods, one at a time, to identify if certain foods trigger behavioral problems.

✓ Artificial food colorings and preservatives will not

cause of ADHD, but may worsen behavior in some children. The elimination diet approach can help determine if this is the case for your child and if these substances should be avoided.

✓ Nutrition management strategies can help counteract the side effect of medications used to treat ADHD, if necessary.

✓ So far, two nutrients have been shown to improve ADHD symptoms: Omega 3 fatty acids and vitamin D.

✓ Behavior management strategies related to nutrition and the food environment are important for all children, especially those with ADHD.

✓ Regular exercise is beneficial for all children for multiple reasons, and can be especially helpful for children with ADHD to improve concentration and attention.

ABOUT THE AUTHOR

Wendy Phillips is a registered dietitian nutritionist with a background in adult and pediatric/infant nutrition support. She has provided nutrition care in a variety of healthcare settings, including home health, hospice, hospitals, long term care, and individual medical nutrition therapy and counseling settings. Her interest in nutrition related to ADHD began when her own son was diagnosed at the age of ten, and she has enjoyed the process of learning with her family and sharing her knowledge with other healthcare professionals and parents of children with ADHD.